Endorsements

"Dr. Khatri incisively describes a dystopian reality that has crept up around us and gutted the doctor-patient relationship. George Orwell and Aldous Huxley would shudder at the keen realization that the narratives contained within Dr. Khatri's book are nonfiction. Readers will enjoy the engaging, colloquial, first-person voice of a caring, empathetic clinician-scientist, which opens our eyes to the insidious force in the examining room."
—Daniel Kantor, MD, FAAN,
Founding President of the Medical Partnership 4 MS (MP4MS),
President Emeritus of the Florida Society of Neurology (FSN) and
Past Chair of Florida Medicaid Pharmacy & Therapeutics Committee

"Dr. Khatri has written a remarkable book. It includes personal, gripping stories about physician burnout and demoralization while practicing medicine in a corporate era–when treatment decisions can be overruled by persons with inadequate medical training; when doctors are fired for expressing concern about quality; when paperwork is given priority over talking with patients. Dr. Khatri tells doctors to fight back, to harness their collective power to change things. He ends with an upbeat message advising colleagues to attend to their own health so that they will have the vigor to engage in the good fight."
—Grace Budrys PhD, author of *Unequal Health* (3rd ed, 2017),
Our Unsystematic Health Care System (4th ed, 2016),
and *When Doctors Join Unions* (1997)

"In this day and age, when time spent on a computer has outpaced time spent with patients; when the only conversation between physician and patient is often 'follow that exit sign to check out,' and when the value of medical care is measured not in healing but in cost, it is not only helpful to understand the causes of a disease that is killing medical providers but also to realize that there may well be a meaningful and effective way of healing the physicians ... Those of us who are privileged to practice medicine would do well to read, reflect on, and become part of the solution to a problem that is escalating out of control."
—Michael P. McQuillen, MD, MA, FAAN,
Former Chairman, Departments of Neurology,
Medical College of Wisconsin, University of Kentucky

"Bhupendra Khatri, in his masterpiece, 'Healthcare 911,' addresses the convergence of a multitude of factors that adversely affect physicians, physician health, and patient care. These include the power and dominance of administrators and the burdens associated with electronic health records, ICD coding, burnout, the Sunshine Act, malpractice, and peer-to-peer

consultations, to name a few. His 'fight-back' message in the form of recommendations is relatively simple: Remain positive, become proactive, play an increased administrative role, help each other, remain patient centric, confront stress with exercise and other healthy choices, and practice kindness (to patients, each other, and yourself). His unwritten final message is abundantly clear. Physicians can, indeed, positively modify the existing patient-care milieu and improve both patient and physician health. The choice is theirs.

—Edward C. Benzel, MD,
Chairman, Department of Neurosurgery, Cleveland Clinic

"This passionate book, written by a dedicated physician, is a wake-up call to all of us that external forces are systematically destroying the patient-physician relationship. Like a biblical prophet warning of impending disaster, Dr. Khatri shows that something is dangerously wrong with a medical system that systematically burns out its most devoted physicians in a fog of electronic health records, complex diagnostic and billing codes, inadequate reimbursements, unjust medical malpractice rules, petty insurance pre-authorization requirements, and diminishing professional prerogatives. He mourns how the business interests of insurance companies, pharmaceutical manufacturers, and hospital systems have squelched physicians' Hippocratic duties to promote patient welfare. His solutions are reasonable, salutary, and urgent."

—James L. Bernat, MD
Professor of Neurology and Medicine (Active Emeritus),
Geisel School of Medicine at Dartmouth

"The ongoing debates about healthcare in the US are dominated by huge industries and government entities; yet rarely does one hear from those who are most directly affected, who daily are engaged on the front lines of healthcare – physicians and their patients. In 'Healthcare 911,' Dr. Khatri gives voice to these constituencies. He melds the observational skills of a master clinician with the gifts of a virtuoso storyteller, bringing vividly (and painfully) to life the toll that our dysfunctional system increasingly is taking on our physicians—and on us as their patients. In his summation, he prescribes what amounts to palliative therapy for his fellow physicians for a malady whose cure must await near total restructuring of our dysfunctional healthcare system."

—Ron Cohen, MD, President and CEO,
Acorda Therapeutics, Inc.

"In an era when physicians are overwhelmed by the electronic medical records, prior authorizations, and a rigid adherence to evidence-based medicine, it is refreshing to read the work of Dr. Khatri—a true neurologist's neurologist. He teaches physicians, both young and experienced, the value of listening carefully to their patients.

"With his deeply personal approach to neurology (and medicine, in general), he follows in the footsteps of William Osler and the late Oliver Sacks. Of late, much has been written about physician burnout. Dr. Khatri's approach to patient care provides practical guidance to keep physicians from losing their way in this fast-changing healthcare environment. He points a way for physicians to sustain themselves as links in the long chain of our noble profession. This book should be on the shelf of every thoughtful physician."

—S. Mitchell Freedman, MD, FAAN. Adjunct Professor of Neurology
UNC Chapel Hill. Raleigh Neurology Associates

"Dr. Khatri is a true thought leader. He accurately describes physicians' changing roles as yoked and buggy-whipped oxen who pull a three-trillion-dollar healthcare industry wagon. To restore their dignity, sanity, and profession, doctors must first admit to themselves they have become assembly-line workers. Then, they must collectively organize to create a more level playing field with employers, insurers, and administrators—for their own sakes as well as their patients'. Thank you, Dr. Khatri, for your insights and courage."

—Stuart Bussey, MD, JD
President, Union of American Physicians and Dentists

"This passionate, well-researched, and well-written book is a thoughtful depiction of current US healthcare and social context. It is clearly the work of a hands-on, caregiving physician and is eminently readable. Its humanity is illustrated by first-person patient and physician stories supported by factual commentary on every aspect of the medical machine. The plight of the doctor, the patient, the medical profession, and society at large, is in sharp focus.

"In this good read, Dr. Khatri has touched on every healthcare aspect. No longer can these issues be ignored or denied. Most importantly, it is a call to arms: Caregiving individuals and organizations are most aware and most prepared for the challenges. It is our responsibility to engage. Reading this book is empowering and is a 'must' for those involved in all aspects of medical care delivery including those who do not provide care at the bedside."

Stephen M. Sergay, MB BCh.
Affiliate Professor of Neurology, University of South Florida
Past president American Academy of Neurology
Founding Chair of the United Council on Neurologic Sub-specialties
Past trustee of the World Federation of Neurology
Managing partner, Tampa Neurology Associates

"Healthcare 911 *is Dr. Khatri's second book. For years, his friends encouraged him to write his stories down. He did this in his first book,* Healing the Soul, *which continues to touch and improve many lives and garner praise from colleagues and patients alike. I was fortunate to have access to the chapters of this new book months before it was published and to witness how it evolved since I first read it.*

"Healthcare 911 *comes at the time of great need when many medical doctors are facing difficult times. Some may feel targeted and persecuted, and yet every single day, they continue to face life-and-death questions on behalf of their patients.* Healthcare 911 *not only poses tough questions about this stressful situation, it also provides thoughtful answers.*

"Dr. Khatri is a true humanitarian, always on the side of those in need. Today, they happen to be his own colleagues. In this new book, he provides us with timely support, arms us with the most powerful tools of kindness and the spirit of giving, and proves to us that we can and will prevail."

—Regina Berkovich MD, PhD
Associate Professor, Dept. of Neurology, USC, LA

HEALTHCARE 911

How America's Broken Healthcare System is
Driving Doctors to Despair,
Depriving Patients of Care, and
Destroying Our Reputation in the World

Other books by Bhupendra O. Khatri

*Healing the Soul: Unexpected Stories of Courage,
Hope, and the Power of Mind*

HEALTHCARE

How America's Broken Healthcare System is
Driving Doctors to Despair,
Depriving Patients of Care, and
Destroying Our Reputation in the World

Bhupendra O. Khatri, MD, FAAN

Hansa House Publishing, LLC
Milwaukee, Wisconsin

Published by
Hansa House Publishing, LLC
www.KhatriMD.com

In collaboration with
HenschelHaus Publishing, Inc.
www.henschelHAUSbooks.com
Milwaukee, Wisconsin

Please contact the publishers for inquiries regarding quantity discounts and special sales to organizations, academic institutions. or other groups.

ISBN: 978159598-594-1
E-ISBN: 978159598-595-8
LCCN: 2018930038

Publisher's Cataloging-In-Publication Data
(Prepared by The Donohue Group, Inc.)

Names: Khatri, Bhupendra O.
Title: Healthcare 911 : how America's broken healthcare system is driving doctors to despair, depriving patients of care, and destroying our reputation in the world / Bhupendra O. Khatri, MD, FAAN.
Description: Milwaukee, Wisconsin : Hansa Publishing, LLC, [2018] | Published in collaboration with HenschelHaus Publishing, Inc. | Includes bibliographical references and index.
Identifiers: ISBN 9781595985941 | ISBN 9781595985958 (ebook)
Subjects: LCSH: Medical care--United States. | Physicians--United States--Interviews. | Health services administration--United States. | Medical policy--United States. | Insurance companies--United States.
Classification: LCC R728 .K43 2018 (print) | LCC R728 (ebook) | DDC 610.68--dc23

This book is dedicated to my physician colleagues.
Your stories made this book.

Contents

Foreword

Healthcare is big business in this country and it is projected to keep growing. The most recent figures released by the Centers for Medicare & Medicaid Services (CMS) indicated, that overall, US spending on healthcare has now reached $3.3 trillion. That amounts to $10,348 per person and 17.9 percent of gross national product (GNP). Medicare, Medicaid, and private insurance expenditures are in the billions.

It's pretty difficult to wrap one's head around those numbers, but when we see words like *billion* and *trillion*, we know we are talking about a lot of money. With a price tag of that size, one would think we must have the best healthcare system in the world; but sadly, we do not. In fact, we are viewed as having one of the *worst* among developed nations.

With our state-of-the-art medical schools, cutting-edge technology, and ground-breaking scientific discoveries, why are we not able to provide adequate healthcare to all of our citizens without sending them into bankruptcy? Why are the prices of prescription drugs soaring, a few as much as 5,000 percent, so that many patients can no longer afford their life-saving medications? And why are American doctors, still in the prime of lives, opting for early-retirement, suffering from stress-related illnesses, and committing suicide in record numbers?

These are only a few of the unanswered questions about what is wrong with the American healthcare system— questions that this book answers from the perspective of besieged physicians. According to Dr. Bhupendra O. Khatri, author of *Healthcare 911*, the delivery of medical services has turned into a high-stakes game, which doctors are surely losing. In fact, the situation has reached crisis proportions.

Not too many years ago, those who entered the field of medicine were held in high esteem—respected, admired, and held up as role models. But that world no longer exists. Today's doctors are stressed, depressed, exhausted, burned out, suffering from a range of illnesses, and having the dubious distinction of the highest rate of suicides of any profession. All of this begs the question, how did this happen?

The issues raised in *Healthcare 911* are only the tip of the iceberg of the problems facing the US healthcare system. If there were a solution on the horizon, Dr. Khatri would have included it in this book. His advice to physicians on how to take better care of themselves is a beginning, but so much more is required. So far, an industrywide solution eludes every player on this uneven playing field. There will be no win -win if things stay the way they are, and the biggest losers will continue to be doctors and their patients. We cannot allow that to happen.

Healthcare 911 is an eloquent, urgent wake-up call to the US medical profession. The problems highlighted in these pages are real, but they are not insurmountable. If you are reading this book, you may have experienced some or all of them. Or, you may be learning about them for the first time. Perhaps you are a member of Congress or the president of an insurance company or a hospital administrator. Whoever you are, whether you are part of the problem or a concerned citizen, you must become part of the solution. Of course, solving this problem is going to take time, innovative thinking, and people power. After reading this book, I want to be part of the solution. I think, after you read it, you will, too.

Joe Sweeney
New York Times Best-Selling Author,
National Speaker, Business & Leadership Consultant,
Businessman, Milwaukee, Wisconsin

Preface

Nearly four-hundred physicians commit suicide each year, and many more simply suffer in silence. Physician burnout has reached dangerous proportions, affecting more than 55 percent of healthcare providers, according to the Mayo Clinic. This is a national healthcare crisis that demands immediate action before it is too late to change its devastating consequences. Spend only one day with your doctor, and you will witness the situation firsthand; read this book, and you will begin to understand the full scope of the problem.

Physicians are being squeezed from every direction: by hospitals and insurance companies that are absorbing private medical practices in unprecedented numbers; by administrators who are interfering with the way doctors care for their patients; and by politicians who pass legislation that benefits corporate entities at the expense of medical providers and patients. Understanding what is really ailing our doctors is the beginning of finding a remedy. To that end, I interviewed hundreds of physicians around the country; their stories burn the pages of this book.

In addition, consider these sobering facts:

- Currently, more than one million patients in the United States lose a physician to burnout, early retirement, or suicide each year.

- By 2030, it is estimated that the American population will surpass 359 million citizens.

- Of those citizens, one in five will be sixty-five or older.

- New primary-care physicians and other medical specialists are not keeping pace with the demands of this growing and aging population.

- In 2030, the country will face a shortage of between 40,800 and 104,900 physicians.

There is no greater problem facing us in the years ahead; it will take a dramatic paradigm shift on the part of all stake-holders to craft a solution. The health of the nation hangs in the balance.

Bhupendra O. Khatri, MD
Milwaukee, Wisconsin

Introduction

There is a little-known healthcare crisis taking place in this country. I am not referring to the recent report by the Commonwealth Fund that the US healthcare system is ranked as the worst in the world among industrialized nations or that an estimated 28 million Americans have no access to healthcare because they are uninsured. The crisis I am talking about is what is happening to our highly educated, well-trained doctors.

Despite the image of competence and confidence they project to their patients, most physicians are working under almost impossible conditions. Their medical practices are being acquired by hospitals, insurance companies, and conglomerates, all of which put profit before patients and exercise absolute control over the business of healthcare.

The result is that physicians are becoming depressed and disillusioned about their ability to properly care for their patients. They are expected to see more patients in less time, while keeping up with voluminous electronic health records, phone calls, and communication through patient portals. They are losing their autonomy, their health, and a good part of their income. Their burnout rate has reached critical proportions. They are retiring early or leaving the field altogether. Essentially, many doctors are dealing with their own silent killer diseases—not immediately apparent but deadly if they are not treated soon.

What precipitated this reversal of the way doctors were viewed and patients were cared for? It doesn't seem so long ago that being a doctor was a prestigious and well-paid profession. Doctors were respected, admired, even revered. They had traveled a long road to become physicians—a road filled with hard work, tough courses, sleepless nights, and many moments when they doubted their ability to make it through. But make it through they did, and the rewards were abundant. Even when house calls and family doctors, who did everything from delivering babies to setting broken bones, were giving way to specialties within specialties, doctors still managed to practice the age-old art of medicine.

Fast forward to the present moment, in which the picture doesn't seem so rosy. The art of medicine is getting lost in a sea of government regulations, corporate demands, and technology that has nothing to do with treating patients. Doctors have always worked hard, but never have they been exhausted in the way they are now. In fact, they are experiencing an unprecedented degree of stress, which is leading many of them to mental and physical collapse.

More than half of US physicians report that they are experiencing burnout. As a matter of fact, doctors are fifteen times more likely to report that they would quit if they could afford to do so. Burnout has consequences. Not only does it affect the quality of physicians' work but their health and personal lives, as well. They have a 10 to 20 percent higher divorce rate than the general population, suffer from stress-induced depression, and are taking their own lives in record numbers. According to www.emedicine.medscape.com, approximately one physician commits suicide every day, making that suicide rate the highest of any profession.

The American medical profession is at a critical juncture, and solving the healthcare juggernaut seems to be beyond the capability of any of the industries involved or Congress, which keeps changing the rules of the game. The critical questions *Healthcare 911* answers are: *How did this situation come about? What are its consequences? And, what can be done to change it?*

How This Crisis Developed

The Patient Protection and Affordable Care Act (ACA), which was signed into law on March 23, 2010, dramatically changed the way physicians practice medicine. Included in the ACA was the mandatory requirement that all physicians use electronic health records (EHR). While this system was supposed to streamline record-keeping and allow hospitals and physicians to communicate with each other, EHR in fact succeeded only in adding another layer of responsibility to the physicians' already demanding schedules.

Hospitals and insurance companies are competing to see who can gain control of primary-care medical practices, which then become referral sources. Within a three-year period, hospitals bought 31,000 physician practices and had 140,000 doctors under their direct control. Not satisfied with only buying private practices, insurance companies increased their holdings by adding hospitals to their portfolios. Remaining an independent practitioner is rapidly becoming financially impossible.

The Consequences for Physicians and Patients

The massive changes that have taken place in medicine in the past few decades have increased doctors' workloads, imposed stricter regulatory requirements, decreased their ability to control their income and the way they care for patients, and intensified their fear of litigation. Taken one at a time, each of these is extremely stressful; together, they are a recipe for job dissatisfaction, depression, burnout, or worse.

As more and more hospitals and insurance companies buy up medical practices, more administrators are hired to oversee and control every aspect of how practices are run. This has created a demanding, hostile work environment for the physicians, who have lost their autonomy and often much more.

Control is something physicians seem to be losing at every turn, particularly when insurance companies deny patient claims for a given medication or therapy. Doctors spend many precious hours in conferences with company-hired doctors, who are in no way peers of the specialists they are talking to and often don't understand either the disease or the recommended therapy. The stated reason for denying a claim is never the real reason; the real reason is profit.

EHRs were supposed to be a boon to doctors and hospitals. Instead, they have become another burden for the medical staff, who are now spending a disproportionate amount of time inputting patients' symptoms, current medications, tests, diagnoses, and prescribed therapies—all in the examining room, with the patient, in the briefest possible amount of time. Among the most aggravating aspects of EHR are the newly mandated International Classification of Diseases (ICD)-10 codes, which turn medical specialists into typists and add significantly to their workloads and stress levels.

Physicians who have worked collaboratively for years with the pharmaceutical industry have been barred by their institutions from continuing with those relationships. The Physicians Payments Sunshine Act (PPSA) didn't actually bar physicians for working with the industry, but the rules and regulations of the law made it very difficult for them to continue to play that role comfortably or to interact with pharmaceutical representatives. This segment of the Affordable Care Act severed not only the mutually beneficial relationship between drug companies and physicians but also eliminated many of medical contributions it produced.

It is no wonder that medical providers worry about litigation instigated by a patient. Malpractice lawsuits can be ruinous to reputations, income, and lives. Even if they are baseless and dismissed in court, their damage can still be felt by doctors who have been sued.

What can be Done to Solve the Problem?

If there were a simple solution, surely someone would have implemented it by now. Over the years, there have been many attempts to reform our broken healthcare system. When Bill Clinton became president, he put his wife in charge of finding the answer. Her attempts to achieve collaboration among the diverse stakeholders involved in healthcare ended in failure. When Barack Obama became president, he outlined his vision for a system that would benefit all involved parties. However, the manner in which the vision was implemented—the Affordable Care Act (ACA)—has not been a resounding success.

The ACA interfered with the patient-physician relationship by attempting to reward physicians who provided "quality" care; telling individual citizens how to purchase their healthcare; and making it necessary for many small employers to change the way they hired employees and managed their operations, with huge penalties imposed by the IRS for non-compliance. The mandatory use of EHR, which was included in the ACA, not only added to physicians' frustration but also further distanced them from their patients.

When Donald Trump became president, he vowed to repeal and replace the ACA, but after seven years of campaigning on that promise, Congress once again ran into a brick wall. The recent drama that took place in Congress over the ACA illustrates the stark reality that healthcare policy in the United States is a political agenda. Consider the following: First, the Republicans refused to work with the Democrats. Second, the Republicans could not agree among themselves on what reform should look. Third, the Republicans, who had the majority in both houses of Congress, ignored the majority of Americans who wanted a practical system that would provide access to decent healthcare services. And since no one has put forth a viable alternative to one of the most complicated and inequitable healthcare systems in the developed world, the hospital, insurance, and pharmaceutical industries continue to reap huge profits, while patients and physicians see their resources dwindling and depleted.

In the course of researching *Healthcare 911*, I interviewed many healthcare providers about how best to deal with this crisis. Their answers would fill another whole book, but here are some particularly practical suggestions offered by a former CEO of a major hospital in the Midwest whom I had the opportunity to interview. This hospital executive, advocated:

1. Establishing public policy that recognizes access to quality healthcare services as a human right of every American.
2. Moving to a single-payer system, whereby all healthcare is purchased (but not run) by the federal government.
3. Requiring that all hospitals and other major healthcare-providers have governing boards that comprise at least 51 percent physicians.
4. Creating a national campaign to promote healthcare as a right so that, over time, we value access to healthcare services no less than we value access to a good education.
5. Providing grants and other types of public funding to competent, well-managed, non-profit organizations that truly still believe that healthcare is a mission.

Imagine a healthcare delivery and financing system based on true competition. The cost of healthcare and insurance premiums would be reduced. Then, all stakeholders would start to make rational economic choices among competing priorities. That might not solve all of the problems we are facing, but it would certainly be good beginning.

Chapter 1
Administrative Power:
A Clear and Present Danger

"Doctors have become worker bees in the factory
of the administrative overload."
—Kevin Campbell, MD, FAAC

During his address at the Mayo Clinic in 1978, Milton Friedman, Nobel laureate and economist, quoted Dr. Gunnar Biörck, a man who was regarded as one of the top heart specialists of the 1970s. Dr. Biörck, the first physician of the Swedish Royal Court, had predicted a "cancerous growth" of hospital administrators in the years ahead. Friedman reiterated that warning, which became reality earlier than he could have foreseen.

Only thirty-eight years later, the Mayo Clinic announced to the world that, based on its extensive research, burnout among US physicians had reached a dangerous level, affecting more than 55 percent of them.

The overwhelming reason cited for this catastrophe is what Dr. Jeff Cain, president-elect of the American Academy of Family Physicians, calls "administrative dominance." By that, he means that hospital administrators directly control most medical practices today. They call the shots, institute new procedures, and push physicians to see more patients in a day, which causes physicians to report feeling like they are running around on a hamster wheel.

1

Not too long ago, physicians took pride in the strenuous and grueling hours they kept. They still work the same hours, but now they are being told by administrators what to do and what not to do, being pressured to see more patients, and asked to follow rigid and senseless regulations that have nothing to do with improving patient care. All of these changes have resulted in increased stress, added clerical duties, work overload, and a dramatic increase in physician burnout over the last three decades. The healers of America are suffering, and unless the cause of this epidemic—the increasing power of hospital and practice administrators—is curtailed, the situation will only get worse.

The following true story exemplifies the rapid and dangerous emergence of administrators who have wreaked havoc on the traditional patient-physician relationship, succeeded in destroying the "healing nature of medicine," and instilled a sense of terror in medical providers, according to the hundreds of physicians with whom I have spoken.

No One is Immune

What recently happened to a world-renowned cardiologist— Dr. Kiran Sagar at the Aurora St. Luke's Medical Center in Milwaukee, Wisconsin—is now happening to other physicians around the country.

Dr. Sagar was the first female cardiologist to practice in the State of Wisconsin. During her thirty years in academic and clinical research, she trained more than 250 cardiologists; published over seventy original research papers in prestigious, peer-reviewed medical journals; contributed chapters to several medical text books; and became internationally recognized for her expertise in echocardiography. Dr. Sagar was passionate about rendering quality care and making her patients' interests her top priority. In 2003, Aurora Health Care hired her to lead its echocardiography and stress-test programs.

While she was covering for a colleague who was away on vacation, Dr. Sagar was asked to perform intraoperative cardiac monitoring (i.e., review and interpret data during surgery). The patient was already on the operating table, anesthetized, on a respirator, and about to undergo open-heart surgery to replace the mitral and aortic valves. As she compared the patient's previous echocardiogram to her own examination, Dr. Sagar realized that she could not corroborate the diagnosis reached by the other cardiologist. Her echocardiogram was entirely normal, a conclusion which she immediately pointed out to the surgeons who were about to operate. The surgery was averted in the nick of time, but this chilling experience led to an epiphany for Dr. Sagar: the error provided a perfect opportunity for research.

Dr. Sagar conducted eighteen months of retrospective study. Her fears were confirmed when she looked at the accuracy of all echocardiograms performed and reported by various cardiologists at her facility. Twenty-nine percent of the echocardiograms had been grossly misread. Recognizing the significance of her findings, the American Society of Echocardiography (ASE) accepted her request to present her findings at its annual national meeting. In her presentation, Dr. Sagar stressed the importance of correct echocardiogram interpretation by trained cardiologists and proposed raising the bar nationally to improve quality of care.

The ASE and the media took notice of her message, as did her hospital administrators. A few months after her groundbreaking presentation, Dr. Sagar was summoned to a meeting with a group of administrators.

"As of now, your employment is terminated," she was told. "We want you to leave the hospital immediately. We will make sure that all your personal belongings are delivered to your home." Shocked, Dr. Sagar asked why.

"We do not have to give you a reason," was the curt reply. "Your contract clearly states that your employment can be terminated without any cause. We further remind you that for another two years, you cannot practice medicine within a twenty-mile radius of this hospital."

Within an hour of the meeting, Dr. Sagar was at home, out of a job. She sat her kitchen table, thinking about what had just happened. Her firing, Dr. Sagar felt, was purely a business decision. Based on the findings of her study, she had wanted to restrict who could read cardiac echoes and, as a result, she fully expected the number of such procedures at her hospital to decline. At age sixty-four, her distinguished thirty-year career was ended abruptly by hospital administrators who seemed to care only about how much money could be made by billing for more procedures performed by physicians.

It did not matter to them what it had taken to build her career: the sacrifices she had made; the battles she had fought to succeed as the only female cardiologist in the entire State of Wisconsin; the lives she had touched and saved; and the research she had done to better serve those with cardiovascular diseases. It all boiled down to money. By allowing only a select group of cardiologists to read echocardiograms, the number of outcomes would result in a tremendous financial loss to the hospital.

Dr. Sagar had always been a fighter. She never bowed to societal pressures and always tried to do what was right. It took a lot of courage to enroll in medical school when only a handful of women at the time were entering the profession. It took a lot of courage as a single woman to leave India and come to the United States and further her education in cardiology. It also took courage to marry an American, who was not only a foot-and-a-half taller than she was but also of different ethnicity and faith.

She remembers carrying *Yellow Pages* telephone books to stand on behind a podium when she presented her research at meetings because the height of the podium was more suited to her male counterparts than to a diminutive woman. "If there is a will, there is a way!" had always been her philosophy.

At the moment, however, she felt numb, violated. Never had she imagined that an administrator in his thirties—who was not even a physician and whose specialty was running the business of medicine—would bring her to her knees. Her situation brought to mind how the Taliban had used a truck-load of dynamite in March 2001 to destroy the world's two largest standing Buddha statues in a matter of minutes. The Buddhas of Bamiyan were fourth- and fifth-century monu-mental statues carved into the side of a cliff in the Bamiyan Valley in central Afghanistan. The Taliban had given no thought to what it had taken to build those statues seventeen hundred years earlier or the significance of what they were doing, just as the hospital administrators who had fired Dr. Sager had thought nothing about the sacrifices it had taken to build her career.

But giving up was not her way. In fact, it had crossed her mind, when she first decided to go public with her research, that the findings of her study might be damaging to the hospital, which took pride in its cardiac care "product line" and was trying to portray itself as one of the leading cardiac centers in the country. It had also occurred to her that she could be putting her job in jeopardy, but she truly believed that the administrators would appreciate the importance of her findings and use them to raise the standards of cardiac care in the hospital, rather than to fire her. Even if the hospital terminated her position, she believed, it could never rob her of her pride, her dignity, or her beliefs. She had no intention of giving in to administrative blackmail.

Dr. Sagar's firing became national news. It was featured in newspapers, *Newsweek* magazine, and on national television. John Fauber, a senior medical reporter for the *Milwaukee Journal Sentinel*, reported that a "cardiologist whose research at a national medical meeting revealed that other doctors at her hospital were misreading a substantial number of diagnostic echocardiograms has been fired by that hospital." In her interview with the same reporter, she said she was never told why she was being let go but suspected it was because of her research on the misread echocardiograms and the publicity that the research generated.

The fact that the administrators were not challenged by any medical organization, even though it was quite clear why Dr. Sagar had been fired, sent a chilling effect throughout the medical community. No matter how competent a physician is or how much research has been done to improve the lives of millions around the world, doctors can be fired on the spot by hospital administrators without being given a reason. No one is immune.

In an email to CNN reporter Marty Makary, an Aurora spokesman said Sagar's firing was not related to her presentation. Makary reported in a special on CNN that, "Dr. Kiran Sagar, a cardiologist in Wisconsin, was fired two months after presenting strong data showing that cardiologists in the hospital at which she worked had misread a substantial number of heart tests." He also reported the case of a nurse from the Columbia Hospital Corporation of America (HCA), "who was let go after complaining that a doctor was performing unnecessary cardiac procedures, even after an internal investigation found the nurse's claim to be substantiated."

Around this time, the CBS News program *60 Minutes* reported that emergency room (ER) doctors were being fired by hospital administrators for not meeting quotas on the percentage of patients they admitted to the hospital. When I asked Dr. Sagar how this all affected her, emotionally, I was troubled by her answer. "What hurt me the most," she said, "was that none of my colleagues spoke up for me against the administrators. They were all afraid for their employment. Speak up, and you risk destroying your career. Administrators have become very powerful."

This is Not Your Father's AMA

Unfortunately, the cancer of which Milton Friedman had warned has come to pass. It has become increasingly common for administrators to fire doctors without expecting any consequences, since physicians are prohibited by the Sherman Antitrust Act from bargaining collectively for their basic rights. This landmark federal statute passed by Congress in 1890 under the Harrison administration allowed certain business activities that were deemed to be competitive and recommended that the federal government investigate and pursue trusts. While the National Labor Relations Act of 1935 (NLRA) gives private-sector employees the right to negotiate collectively with their employers, hospital-employed physicians who wish to do so must meet stringent requirements. The US Federal Trade Commission (FTC) and the US Department of Justice (DOJ) continue to actively enforce the antitrust laws with respect to hospitals, doctors, and others in the healthcare field.

The American Medical Association (AMA) was created in 1847 to preserve and protect the interests of physicians. Now, it is widely regarded by the medical community as being impotent. Only 17 percent of US doctors are members of the AMA. According to a recent Jackson & Coker (a physician recruiter) industry survey, an astonishing 77 percent of physicians don't think the AMA represents their interests. However, despite its dwindling membership, the AMA thrives on the billing codes it has created, known as Current Procedural Terminology (CPT). These mandated billing codes add to the administrative duties physicians must perform, while the association earns in excess of $70 million a year in royalties.

The significance of what is now happening in medical care is profound. One in four doctors in the United States will reach retirement age in five years. One in three doctors is over fifty; one in four is over sixty; there are not enough new doctors being trained to meet the medical needs of Americans. According to a 2013 survey of over twenty thousand physicians by the health division of Deloitte, the largest consulting firm in the world, 62 percent say "it is likely that many physicians will retire earlier than planned in the next one to three years, mainly because of the increasingly unnecessary and mandatory demands being put on them."

The world population has doubled in the last fifty years from three billion to six billion. By 2050, it is expected to reach nine billion. In the United States, population is projected to grow by 89 million residents from 2010 to 2050. The population of seniors in this country will more than double, from 41 to 86 million. Medical needs will increase exponentially. As the projected physician shortage puts our nation in crisis mode, ironically, the number of healthcare administrators is dramatically increasing. In contrast to a less than one percent per year net growth in the number of physicians entering the workforce, there has been a 3,000 percent increase in healthcare administrators over the last three decades (Young et al, *Journal of Medical Regulation*, 2017).

The Compensation Crisis

Why such a dramatic rise? What does this mean to physicians and their practice of medicine? What does it mean to patients in terms of added cost for their medical care? The answers to these questions are disturbing. Increasing regulations have necessitated more administrators to oversee and enforce them. Whereas once only a few such professionals were required, and doctors were in charge of their medical practices, that old model has been turned upside down. As hospitals have continued to buy up private practices, administrators have grown not only in number but also in power. In a stunning role reversal, they are now the ones who are running the show, rather than the physicians. In essence, administrators are controlling every aspect of the healthcare system.

Currently, the base pay of hospital executives and hospital administrators outstrips doctors' salaries, according to an analysis performed by Compdata Surveys for *The New York Times*. The median salary for a hospital CEO is $386,000 and $237,000 for a hospital administrator, compared with $306,000 for a surgeon and $185,000 for a general practitioner. According to *The New York Times*, "Physicians, the most highly trained members in the industry's workforce, are not the top earners. On average, they are right in the middle of the compensation pack. That is because the biggest bucks are currently earned not through the delivery of care, but from overseeing the business of medicine."

According to an article in www.NJBIZ.com, "Medical Millionaires: The Compensation Packages of Hospital Heads Are Drawing Attention," Joseph Trunfio, CEO of the three-hospital Atlantic Health System in Morristown, New Jersey, received a total cash compensation of $10.7 million in 2012, a 201.9 percent increase over his prior year's compensation. William Petasnick, CEO of Milwaukee-based Froedtert Health, received $6.6 million in total compensation in 2012, a 227.2 percent hike from 2011. Studies suggest that administrative costs make up 20 to 30 percent of the US healthcare bill. Actually, 1.43 percent of the US GDP of $18,570 billion US dollars in 2016, or $266 billion, was spent on hospital administration costs. This is expected to rise to $315 billion in 2018, according to Dr. Sara R. Collins, a Commonwealth Fund economist, with an inverse relationship between administrative costs and quality of care. As administrators continue to earn more, physicians see their income declining, and patients watch their costs rising to cover administrative salaries.

While the cumulative increase in the inflation rate over the last decade was 10 percent, our own medical practice at the Center for Neurological Disorders saw a decline in revenue of 20 percent, even though the number of patients seen in the clinic had not decreased. This is not an isolated incident, but a national trend. As doctors lose control of their clinics and compensation with the implementation of the ACA, they are forced to give up their independence and to become employed by hospital systems. Federal health laws, policies adopted by hospital administrators, and the ever-increasing restrictions implemented by medical-insurance companies make it very difficult for independent physicians to survive.

At best, administrators do what they are trained to do: administer the practice of medicine as a business. This is contrary to the what physicians are trained to do: choose the most appropriate medical therapies for their patients, regardless of how much money the hospital will earn. Hospitals are buying up private practices at a rate not seen since the late 1990s. A survey conducted in 2011 by the Medical Group Management Association showed that almost 75 percent more doctors have been employed by hospitals since 2000, compared to the early 1990s.

Even more frightening is the acquisition of clinics by health insurance companies—much like the proverbial fox guarding the chicken coop! To save money, these companies offer bonuses to physicians for ordering fewer tests and prescribing the least-expensive medications. While there are no studies that reveal the consequences of this practice, it doesn't take a genius to predict them. The most likely outcomes would be to force doctors to see more patients in less time, drastically curtail necessary tests, and attach more importance to saving money than to taking care of patients.

This is not only an ethical issue but also a good example of how administrators are interfering with the practice of medicine. While private practices are declining in number, clinics controlled by larger corporations are rapidly increasing. This trend is doing irreparable damage to the way patients are treated in this country. For one thing, it is obvious that individual physicians know their patients better than large corporations do. For another, large corporations have a system for filling their ranks. Primary-care doctors are the first to be hired, which secures firm control over patient referrals to specialists. Next hired are the specialists, who are expected to see a large number of patients per day, follow the rules put in place by the administrators, and accept slashed year-end bonuses for which they are given no valid reason. They are also at risk of being fired without cause, which intensifies an already stressful work environment.

Many doctors and nurses have confided in me about how hospital administrators coerced them into writing derogatory letters about their colleagues that could later be used as evidence for firing those individuals. At first, it sounded absurd to me that this kind of practice existed, but I have since experienced it firsthand! Frightened for their own job security, some physicians give in and do write such letters, pointing out some "faults" they may have noticed in their fellow physicians.

Recently, I visited a group of physicians in Portland, Oregon, who had been hired by a hospital. What they told me was not only shocking but, sadly, not at all unusual.

Their demanding schedule begins at 7:00am, when they look over laboratory results and MRIs. Shortly after that, the clinic begins, with patients who need urgent attention often added to an already long list of patients to see.

The physicians in this group work through their lunch hours, see patients again in the afternoon, and then return patient calls. Even though the clinic ends at 4:00pm, they rarely leave the office before 6:30. After spending some time at home with their families, they put in an extra hour or two before they finally call it a day. For all of the work they do, these physicians are financially compensated only for the actual face-to-face time they spend with their patients.

Another new demand entails communicating with patients through online portals. If patients' questions are not answered promptly, they pile up in electronic in-baskets (like your private email inbox), which is considered bad business practice and can lead to disciplinary actions or curtailing of year-end bonuses. This portal service, according to administrators, generates great marketing dividends for the hospital; unfortunately, it pays no dividends to the physicians. In fact, after three warnings to clean up their in-baskets and medical records, physicians can be fired or have their clinical privileges suspended.

I inquired about why physicians don't object to this punishing schedule or refuse to work for more than their equivalent of "full-time employment hours." Their response was unanimous: "Squeaky wheels get fired by the administrators. Besides, we were made to sign a two-year, non-compete clause. Uprooting the family is not easy, and the grass is no greener on the other side."

This practice has led to demoralization and burnout among physicians across the country, which are now at a record high. To exert their power and ensure their own financial well-being, I was told that administrators systematically weed out physicians who are well known and command respect in their communities. Dr. Robert Abrams's (not his real name) story supports this most recent practice.

Dr. Abrams, a Midwest-based cardiologist, who was regarded by his peers as one of the best in the field, became a victim of hospital administrative dominance. Soon after completing his fellowship, Dr. Abrams was recruited by a large, private cardiology practice. Hard work, compassion, and consistently good clinical outcomes made him one of the most sought-after interventional cardiologists in the state. He was loved and trusted by his peers, staff, and patients.

He began work at 6:30 in the morning and stayed until 7:00pm, five days a week, often working weekends, as well. His group of physicians dominated cardiology care in the city. Important research and excellent patient care earned his institution a reputation as one of the leading cardiology centers in the nation. Dr. Abrams became the hospital's poster child and was featured in newspapers, on billboards, and in television commercials. However, this did not last long.

Eventually, the hospital made an offer to hire Dr. Abrams' cardiology group as a whole, rather than just individual physicians within the group. This created a dilemma because most of the practice's referrals came from primary-care doctors who had already been hired by the hospital system. If Dr. Abrams and his colleagues turned down the offer, the hospital would simply hire other cardiologists to replace them. With both primary care doctors and cardiologists now on the staff, it was logical to assume all referrals would be made to in-house physicians.

Feeling that they had no choice, the doctors accepted the offer. There were no problems during the first few years of their employment, but then things changed. The hospital administrators began to pressure physicians to see more patients in less time, restricting the days they were allowed to take off, cutting down the number of nurses and mid-level providers, and decreasing year-end bonuses. Even though the group had signed a ten-year contract, renegotiations took place every year, always ending in the hospital's favor.

Financial compensation for physicians is based on relative value units (RVUs), Medicare's reimbursement formula for measuring the value of physicians' services. RVUs are dependent upon three key factors: the number of patients seen by the physician, the cost of doing business or maintaining a practice, and the malpractice or liability expenses borne by the provider. Each RVU has a dollar value that is spelled out in the physician's contract. A tactic commonly employed by hospital administrators is to arbitrarily reduce compensation due to a "change in RVUs and the need to stay within the standard fair market value," which varies from city to city and the demand for certain specialties.

Since there is no fixed amount assigned to RVUs, they can be manipulated or reduced by the hospital. Opposition to this reduction by any member of a physician group could result in that person's termination. By using the age-old tactic of "divide and conquer," administrators will either force the rest of the group to accept the new terms or hire new physicians who do not require the same level of financial compensation. An added incentive for new recruits is the promise of more patients, which would increase the number of RVUs earned by the newly hired physician.

Hospitals make money from procedures ordered by physicians; therefore, increasing the number of employed physicians also increases the number of procedures. According to Dr. Abrams, instead of receiving assistance with his extremely busy schedule, patients who should have been referred to him were now being diverted to other physicians. As a result, his income was slashed by fifty percent. This was the last straw for Dr. Abrams. He left the practice, uprooted his family, took his children out of school, and moved to another state, where he built a new practice from scratch.

Who were the losers in this situation? The answer is everyone. Wisconsin lost a great cardiologist. The hospital lost a popular doctor who had helped to build the institution's reputation. But the biggest losers, by far, were Dr. Abrams's patients who loved him, trusted him, and received exceptional care from him.

Increased Demands on Doctors

A short while ago, I was in Spokane, Washington, and had a chance to meet some of the local neurologists who were employed by a hospital that had been acquired by an even bigger corporate entity. The new administrators learned of the three-month waiting period for prospective new patients to see a neurologist. To them, this was an unacceptable business practice. A specially appointed administrator was soon able to fix the problem by insisting that physicians double-book patients! When he heard that, one of the staff neurologists became furious and lashed out at the administrator. "If you want me to double book, give me a double-decker exam room, so I can examine both patients at the same time!" Then, he abruptly left the room. That ridiculous double-booking "solution," which solved nothing, put additional pressure on doctors and forced patients to wait an hour to see doctors who, obviously, could not see twice the number of patients in the allotted time.

In addition to an increased patient load, physicians are routinely pressured to be sure that patient satisfaction surveys are favorable. If they are not, the value of RVUs earned is reduced. Years of training and experience attach no additional value to what a physician can bill or the worth of RVUs in his or her specialty. It is ironic, therefore, that the drastic increases in salaries of CEOs and administrators of not-for-profit hospitals are "well justified" based on the "value" they bring to those hospitals.

It is doctors and other healthcare professionals who make hospitals great. Patients go to a particular medical center because of its doctors, not because of its administrators. I have yet to find a patient who cites an administrator as the reason for choosing a particular clinic or hospital. In fact, patients hate some of the requirements put in place by administrators. They complain about the excessive and repetitive information required at each new visit. "It is all in your computers," they say with frustration. Some complain of spending more time "filling out forms" than they do with their doctors. But each of the encounters with the patient by any member of medical or nursing staff is billable to insurance companies and is, therefore, a revenue generator. It is common knowledge that, as far as administrators are concerned, this repetitive information gathering outweighs any inconvenience reported by patients.

Administrators are beginning to recognize that it is, indeed, doctors who attract patients, but that is not where they want the emphasis to be. Many of them have changed their advertising tactics to effectively shift the limelight from doctors to "programs" or "product lines" offered at their hospitals and clinics. They now tend to promote hospitals and their special programs, rather than physicians, because it is a "bad business decision" to invest in someone who may become a "competitor" if the doctor is hired by another hospital.

Of course, there is always a non-compete clause that physicians are required to sign at the beginning of their employment. This practically bars them from practicing medicine in areas surrounding the hospital (usually, a twenty-mile radius) for at least two years after the termination of their employment. For physicians, this clause is difficult to challenge in court; large corporations have deep pockets and can drag out a lawsuit as long as necessary. Being prevented from working during that time puts the physician at a distinct disadvantage.

The same group I met with in Spokane told me how they are overworked and seriously in need of an additional neurologist to better serve their community. Neurologists are in great demand and not easy to recruit. According to a study published by Thomas R. Vidic, MD, "There is a now a long wait for patients to see a neurologist, and it is difficult to find neurologists to fill vacant positions. In addition, the demand for neurologists is expected to grow as people gain coverage through healthcare reform."

Fortunately, a couple (made up of two physicians) was moving to Spokane. The husband, an oncologist, had already been recruited by an oncology group; his wife, a neurologist, was still looking for a job. The wife came with great qualifications and perfect references; she was exactly what the neurology group at the hospital was looking for. She agreed with everything the hospital had to offer—except that she did not want to sign a non-compete clause. The hospital administrators would not budge, despite persistent appeals from their doctors. As a result, the neurologist was not hired. This was obviously a business decision rather than a healthcare decision.

On the other hand, these same hospitals splash the message on TV and billboards that they are all about people and their needs. Some even have a trademarked slogan proclaiming their patient-centered philosophy.

Physicians are not the only ones targeted by administrators; well-trained and experienced nurses who command higher salaries are also fair game. They are being replaced by younger, less-experienced nurses to cut expenses. More and more is demanded of those who stay, driving them to the point of breakdown. An article titled, "Hospitals Firing Seasoned Nurses: Nurses FIGHT Back!" made the point that "the hospital takes better care of administration than it does of the staff caring for patients."

Practicing Medicine in the Age of Mega-Mergers

Hospital mega-mergers are yet another cancer that has invaded the healthcare delivery system. These mergers are on the rise and are rapidly changing the landscape of the healthcare industry. They grant hospitals enormous market leverage to drive up healthcare costs. What is the real reason for mergers? Are they for the benefit of top executives and shareholders, or do they benefit consumers as well? There is still a lack of consensus among experts about their long-term impact on patient care, but a few of the hospital mergers that have been investigated by the Federal Trade Commission (FTC) revealed that patients were being shortchanged.

One conclusion is obvious: consumers now have limited choices, while hospitals command a monopoly and, thus, can drive up the costs of the services they offer.

According to Barak Richman, JD, PhD, a professor of law and business administration at Duke University, "It is important to note that, once mergers occur, it is very difficult to undo them. Healthcare costs continue to rise—despite mergers—at a financially unsustainable level." Richman called the situation a "national crisis."

In the Boston area, a merged healthcare institution was investigated; the findings support the hypothesis that mergers, in fact, do not lower healthcare costs. The institution demanded high reimbursements from insurers, unrelated to the quality or complexity of care delivered.

Mergers also adversely affect staff and physicians. The hospital at which I work—St. Francis Hospital in Milwaukee—is one of many hospitals owned by Wheaton Franciscan Healthcare (WFHC). Just a few months ago, Ascension Health (AH), the world's largest Catholic healthcare system, announced that it had reached an agreement to add WFHC's Southeastern Wisconsin business to their organization.

"WFHC and AH share the same mission—caring for all persons, especially those who are struggling the most," said Robert J. Henkel, FACHE, executive vice president of Ascension and president and CEO of AH. "We share the same approach to serving our communities—providing compassionate, personalized care to all throughout their lives." It was reported in the *Milwaukee Journal Sentinel* that the reasons for the merger were to better align WFHC and Columbia St. Mary's Hospital. The reason was to better compete with Aurora Health Care, the state's largest healthcare system, and to meet the changing landscape of the health-insurance market and the way doctors and hospitals are paid for their services.

It remains to be seen how this is going to pan out, but I do know that several layers of administrators have already been appointed, and the effects are apparent. Many staff members who have worked at our hospital for years received severance notices. One employee, who had been in the media department for more than twenty-four years, had hoped to retire from this hospital. Instead, he got a termination notice. He was at a loss as to what to do next at his age. He is not quite old enough to retire and not quite young enough to be favorably hired by another company. He approached me for a letter of recommendation, which I wrote with a heavy heart because of countless other people I know at WFHC who were also similarly affected by this huge "successful merger."

We run one of the largest multiple sclerosis (MS) clinics in the country, caring for more than four thousand patients. MS strikes patients in the prime of their lives; it is a lifelong, disabling disease with no cure. As a result, patients with MS suffer from significant psycho-social issues. A social worker in our department was a godsend for these patients. She had done a phenomenal job, allowing us to see more patients in our clinic. Without her, we would be compelled to address their social as well as medical issues, requiring considerably more time with each patient and taking us away from other patients who also need neurological attention. It is not an exaggeration to say that she saved many lives with her interventions, ensuring that patients got prompt psychological help if they were suicidal, had adequate food, and were not abused. In short, she contributed much to the welfare of our patients.

Unfortunately, the new administration did not see things this way. Social-service care is not billable and, inasmuch as the new administration did not see our social worker bringing in revenue on paper, it may not have understood the hidden value she brought to our patients. She received her termination notice while she was away on vacation. We wrote a letter to the hospital CEO, explaining the importance of our social worker to our patients. The hospital agreed to rehire her on the condition that we fire one of the secretaries to make up for the additional salary. Morale, of course, was dashed. On August 5, 2016, headlines in the business section of the *Milwaukee Journal Sentinel* read "Ascension Silent on Job Losses." The paper did not follow up on this article. Not only Ascension but also the media have been silent on reporting the consequences of job losses.

The Ultimate Cost

All of these recent changes contribute to stress and dissatisfaction among physicians, young and old. A record number of physicians is retiring prematurely. With a decreasing pool of active doctors, delivery of healthcare will suffer in the years to come. Not only are reimbursements under the ACA much lower than reimbursements under Medicare but there is also an increasing demand that physicians must care for more patients. Already under significant stress, many physicians have no choice but to take on additional patients to make up for lost revenue. This, in turn, puts more stress on them, creates a vicious cycle, and, eventually leads to physician burnout.

A neurologist who practiced in Tennessee for twenty-five years is one of the many victims of this crisis. Being the only neurologist within a fifty-mile radius, he was on call seven days a week. He treated patients with stroke, headaches, seizures, and many other conditions. He provided evaluation and care when primary-care doctors needed help. He recalled the last five years as "very difficult." Overhead costs were going up, more staff was needed to keep up with added administrative work, a significant and mandatory financial investment in electronic health records (EHR) software had to be made, an ever-increasing need to get authorization from insurance companies was required, reimbursement for his services decreased, and malpractice insurance costs increased. All of this left him with no choice but to give up his private practice. He considered premature retirement but, for financial reasons, he had to work. Rather than being hired by a large hospital corporation to be a "worker bee" (in his words), he joined a Veterans Administration (VA) hospital.

He told me he had been "forced out of (his) private practice and felt like a broken man." He never imagined ending his satisfying and well-respected career this way. Uprooted from friends and a community where they had deep roots, he and his family were forced to live thousands of miles away in the Midwest.

"The first bitter cold winter was extremely difficult. Not having driven in snow before, it was a challenge. I need to work for ten more years, and then we are out of here!" he says. He is not a happy man, and yet, he feels proud that he did not sell his soul to corporate America.

Many other physicians are simply giving up and retiring prematurely. Recent surveys by both Harvard University and the physician recruiting firm, Merritt Hawkins & Associates, produced similar findings: Nearly 40 percent of physicians over age fifty are retiring or actively thinking about it; 12 percent are considering changing careers. Doctors no longer enjoy the autonomy and control they once did. They can handle hard work, as they have done for hundreds of years. It is the manner in which they are now asked to work that is tearing them apart. They see the workplace atmosphere as "negative" and feel that it is having an adverse effect on their minds and bodies.

Extra work done with positive energy never hurts. When doctors meet and reminisce about the work they did during the "good old days" (and the conversation always turns to this), I am surprised by how upbeat they are, even though the number of hours they worked then was much the same as the time they are putting in now. The major difference is that, in those days, they got so much satisfaction out of their work that it didn't matter how hard or how long they worked. They had a close bond with their patients and their patients' families and were not constantly being watched and harassed by administrators or insurance companies. Even though they returned home late every day, they felt satisfied and happy, knowing they were making a difference.

Practicing medicine was an enriching experience for them. In fact, this positive energy nurtured their bodies and souls. It made them proud of what they did. According to motivational speaker Steve Pavlina, "Hard work is painful when life is devoid of purpose. But when you live for something greater than yourself and the gratification of your own ego, then hard work becomes a labor of love."

More Administrators, More Real Estate to House Them

Twenty-five years ago, the few administrators we had at the hospital in which I worked were housed in six rooms. Now, they need a large, free-standing corporate building to accommodate their rising numbers. Recently and for the first time, I visited the corporate building of the healthcare system we now work with; I was amazed by how big the building was. This is not unique to Milwaukee. It is the same story nationwide. Administrators enjoy huge office suites, while physicians have to make do with tiny, windowless workspaces.

One would assume that this growth would be indicative of patient and physician satisfaction; however, it turns out that this relationship is inversely related. Across the country, doctors are frustrated by administrative dominance. The burden of the costs that sustain an army of administrators is eventually passed on to patients. The cost of medical services—not physicians' fees—has risen sharply over the last two decades. Ultimately, all of this affects the care rendered to patients. Based on multiple surveys, patient satisfaction has dropped sharply in the recent years.

In his report in the *Wisconsin State Journal*, David Wahlberg, editor and publisher of the nonprofit *Georgia Health News*, explored the healthcare system in Wisconsin with an emphasis on consumers. This report was triggered by a complaint raised by Dr. Hans Rechsteiner, a general surgeon practicing in rural Wisconsin. Dr. Rechsteiner noted that the hospital bill for an appendectomy for one of his patients was $12,500, more than seven times his fee of $1,700 for doing the surgery. Other charges included $4,000 for the operating room, $3,000 for anesthesia, and $2,500 for the recovery room—all for what Dr. Rechsteiner said was a fifteen-minute procedure. We often laugh at jokes such as "How many electricians does it take to change a light bulb?" Well, do you know how much it costs to administer two tablets of Tylenol to a hospital patient? Brace yourself! One of my patients actually showed me her hospital bill, which listed that cost at $30!

Dr. Rechsteiner and his colleagues in Northern Wisconsin decided it was time to speak out against rising medical costs and get the attention of lawmakers and statewide medical organizations. In a half-page advertisement in the *Wisconsin State Journal*, they called for shutting down of some overbuilt hospitals. They further recommended that patient deductibles should be set as a percentage of total bills, not at a particular amount, so that patients would have more incentive to shop around.

A healthcare administrator, who was a CEO of a hospital in the Midwest in the 1980s, made some insightful comments during my recent communication with him. "Why is it that, before a physician is allowed to care for the life and health of a patient," he asked, "you have to undergo years of education and training and then earn a license before you can practice? However, in order to run a hospital (which is where the physician heals the patient), you literally need no formal education, training, or license. Yet, as an administrator," he pointed out, "you wield a great deal of power over the physician who is caring for the patient. Maybe healthcare administrators should be required to undertake extensive training, with special emphasis on ethics and humanities, and become licensed only if they demonstrate proficiency as individuals who will always be mindful of their duty to care for patients."

This former administrator is very concerned about the rising power of those who now hold these positions. During the time he functioned as a CEO, doctors sat at the table and made all decisions related to patient care, while administrators were asked to take seats on the sidelines, with instructions to speak only if invited to by the chief of the medical staff, who chaired those meetings. This power, held by physicians to make all decisions related to patient care, was sacred until the early 1980s. The last three decades have seen a dramatic shift in that power to administrators. Now, it is physicians who sit on the periphery and await an invitation to speak by those in charge.

More to ACA than Meets the Eye

Now that the implications of the ACA are realized, the concerns raised by Dr. Rechsteiner and his colleagues resonate very well with physicians. Under the ACA, more people now have insurance but very little is done to address soaring healthcare costs, adequate reimbursement for clinic visits, and the physician-burnout crisis. Doctors are now forced to see more patients in a day in order to pay for overhead, while still trying to run a profitable business. This, in turn, leads not only to mental and physical fatigue but also to an increase in therapeutic errors.

I recently interviewed a physician who had been rated a "Top Physician" in Milwaukee for three years in a row. He cared for his patients and took pride in his profession, but now, he is "simply frustrated."

"I never imagined myself having to put up with all this garbage that is thrown at us. I have had it with everyone telling me what to do and forcing me to comply with all of the regulations! Frankly, I have given up!" he lamented. "I simply do what I am asked to do. I am not a physician to my patients anymore. I am made to act like a robot, a computer pusher! Gone are the days when I could afford to hold my patient's hand and sympathize because her spouse of fifty years had just died."

Alas, our pain is felt and recognized by Dr. Vivek Murthy, former US Surgeon General. In 2016, he said, "The suicide and burnout rate is very high, and this is concerning to me because we're at a point in our country where we need more physicians, not fewer; we need more people entering our profession, not fewer. If we have people burning out, it really goes against our needs."

Chapter 2
Electronic Health Records:
Breakthrough or Barrier
to Patient Care?

"Tellingly, the more advanced the EHR (e.g., systems that offer reminders,
alerts, and messaging capability), the greater the unhappiness."
—Robert Wachter, (author of *The Digital Doctor:*
Hope, Hype, and Harm at the Dawn of Medicine's Computer Age)

According to Dr. Steven J. Stack, an emergency physician with a special expertise in health-information technology and the youngest elected president of the American Medical Association (AMA) since 1854, "Electronic health records (EHR) have been essentially reduced to a tool for billing, compliance, and litigation that also has a sustained negative impact on doctors' productivity. Documenting a full clinical encounter in an EHR is pure torment." This is exactly how the majority of the physicians in this country also feel about EHR.

On February 17, 2009, Congress signed into law a $787 billion American Recovery and Reinvestment Act, which included $19.2 billion to be used to increase the use of EHR by physicians and hospitals. This portion of the bill, called the Health Information Technology for Economic and Clinical Health (HITECH) Act, represents the largest US initiative to make the use of EHR by physicians compulsory. Penalties of up to 5 percent reduction in Medicare payments would be imposed on doctors who failed to implement EHR by 2015.

Within a very short time, the law changed the way doctors practice medicine in this country. If the early results of large-scale physician surveys are correct and predictive, this trend could well lead to the demise of the art of practicing of medicine, which took centuries to develop. With EHR, we are experimenting with an unproven, yet mandatory, technology at a national level. No other industry has ever been forced to comply with a new technology before its effects are fully studied. Physicians across the nation fear the wheels that have been set in motion would be difficult to stop, let alone reverse, the damage that is already taking place.

The Centers of Medicare and Medicaid define EHR as follows on the www.cms.gov website:

> "An Electronic Health Record (EHR) is an electronic version of a patient's medical history, that is maintained by the provider over time, and may include all of the key administrative clinical data relevant to that person's care under a particular provider, including demographics, progress notes, problems, medications, vital signs, past medical history, immunizations, laboratory data and radiology reports. The EHR automates access to information and has the potential to streamline the clinician's workflow. The EHR also has the ability to support other care-related activities directly or indirectly through various interfaces, including evidence-based decision support, quality management, and outcomes reporting.

> EHRs are the next step in the continued progress of healthcare that can strengthen the relationship between patients and clinicians. The data, and the timeliness and availability of it, will enable providers to make better decisions and provide better care. For example, the EHR can improve patient care by:

- Reducing the incidence of medical error by improving the accuracy and clarity of medical records.

- Making the health information available, reducing duplication of tests, reducing delays in treatment, and keeping patients well informed to make better decisions.

- Reducing medical error by improving the accuracy and clarity of medical records."

What Do Physicians Think of EHR?

Data released in 2014 by the marketing and research firm MPI Group and Medical Economics suggest that 79 percent of one thousand doctors surveyed had very negative opinions of EHR. They felt implementation of EHR in their offices was not worth the cost, and the majority of respondents said their EHR systems resulted in financial losses. The outcomes of this two-year study are further corroborated by an earlier 2013 RAND Corporation study, detailed in *Health Affairs*, *The New York Times*, and *USA Today*.

According to this survey, "Poor EHR usability, time-consuming data entry, interference with face-to-face patient care, inefficient and less-fulfilling work content, inability to exchange health information between EHR products, and degradation of clinical documentation were prominent sources of professional dissatisfaction." Healthcare providers are now forced to bring computers into examination rooms and type in the patient's symptoms and physical findings, order the necessary tests and treatment plans, and complete all of this in less than forty-five minutes for a new patient and under twenty minutes for a follow-up visit. Something had to give for this "meaningful use of EHR"—a term coined by lawmakers in

Washington, DC—to succeed. Sad to say, what "gave" were the feelings of comfort and trust between doctors and their patients. Often, physicians were so intent on typing that they forgot to look up. Patients felt discounted; physicians felt stressed. It was a lose-lose scenario.

Change, I am told, is good. Change leads to progress. The medical field has seen and embraced remarkable scientific advances over the years to prolong survival and improve quality of life. The driving force behind almost all medical advances has been the sage, old saying, "Necessity is the mother of invention." On the other hand, pushing an agenda before its time can lead to disastrous outcomes. The United States leads the world in medical innovation. Most recent medical breakthroughs have occurred in this country. We have the best and brightest people practicing medicine in state-of-the-art facilities. Patients come from all over the world to access the latest medical technologies and discoveries. This unprecedented progress has occurred despite any agenda set by legislators.

Three of our senses—sight, hearing, and touch—are the physician's most effective diagnostic tools, and speech is our best therapeutic means. To accurately diagnose a medical problem, we must observe the patient, listen to her complaints, and finally examine her. In neurology, we are taught not to touch the patient until we have narrowed our possible diagnoses down to a few, based on taking her medical history and simply observing her. Physical examination and ancillary tests are then performed to confirm our initial impression. Mistakes occur when physicians have no time to listen to or observe the patient. This is what happened to my patient, Hilda.

The Danger of an Incorrect Diagnosis

While she was at work, Hilda, a fifty-six-year-old woman, experienced weakness on the left side of her body; a moment later, she collapsed to the floor. An ambulance came within minutes; an EMT assessed her and radioed the emergency room to announce that they would be bringing in a patient with a possible stroke. When Hilda arrived at the community hospital, an ER physician quickly examined her before sending her for a CT scan of her brain. The radiologist called ER to say that the brain looked normal.

Since there had been no improvement in her weakness, the ER doctor became concerned and called a major hospital some one hundred miles away to discuss his patient, whom he thought might be a good candidate for tissue plasminogen activator (tPA), a protein involved in the breakdown of blood clots. A stroke occurs when a clot cuts off blood flow to parts of the brain. If the blood flow is not resumed within hours, the brain tissue will be permanently destroyed. tPA dissolves clots and restores blood flow. This most dramatic and revolutionary improvement in the care of stroke patients was approved by the FDA some twenty years ago. Stroke used to rank fourth in leading causes of death in this country, but due to advances in medical treatment, it has slipped to fifth. This therapy, however, has potential complications. The chief risk is intracerebral hemorrhage, which occurs in about 6 percent of patients. When this happens, close to half of them die. Other less frequent complications include bleeding elsewhere in the body.

Only after the doctor was able to enter all the details into her EHR was Hilda flown in an ambulance helicopter to a larger hospital. The receiving doctor at this major hospital reviewed the previous ER physician's notes. Hilda's history and the recorded examination was consistent with a "classic stroke," making her a good candidate for tPA. The doctor did a quick examination, reviewed her EHR to make sure there were no contraindications, and then proceeded to give her tPA.

Hilda tolerated the tPA well and had no side effects. The following morning, it was my turn to see all of the in-patients in the hospital. I stopped by the ICU to see Hilda for the first time. She was still unable to move the left side of her body. As I spent more time talking to her, I started to have some doubts about her diagnosis. Had she really had a stroke? My neurological examination further strengthened my doubts. I ordered an MRI scan of her brain, which was completely normal. This confirmed my clinical suspicion that Hilda had not had a stroke. In my opinion, she was suffering from a psychosomatic disorder.

What "Psychosomatic" Really Means

"Psychosomatic disorders" occur when stress causes or aggravates a physical condition. Emotional overload, especially if it goes on for some time, switches on the nervous, endocrine, and immune systems. In response to a threat or stress, a series of events occur in order, starting with the amygdala, hypothalamus, pituitary, and adrenal glands. This is known as "fight or flight" response, in which the sympathetic nervous system produces three major stress hormones—adrenaline, cortisol, and norepinephrine.

All of this puts the body into a state of alertness, which is not healthy. These abnormal physiological changes caused by stress affect virtually all of the body's organs and can lead to psychosomatic illnesses, such as a heart attack, cancer, or an infection. While the symptoms that mimic these illnesses are real, they are not due to actual disorders that affect related organs. Psychological stress, for example, can cause chest pains (without anything really being wrong with the heart) or weakness or paralysis (without anything being wrong with the brain) or severe abdominal pains (without anything being wrong with the organs in the abdomen).

The stress doesn't have to be external; it could be internal. Patients with psychosomatic illnesses seek medical help for their physical symptoms, rather than for emotional stress or trauma. In fact, they are often unaware of the underlying problem.

Emotional trauma or stress may show up as a physical disability. Because there are no obvious abnormalities in the brain or other parts of the body that can explain these symptoms, doctors often order multiple, repetitive tests. Hilda's diagnosis was a stroke, but if one of those doctors had examined her more carefully, he might have noticed the telltale signs of a psychosomatic disorder.

When I first examined Hilda, she complained of complete paralysis of her left arm, yet the position of her arm of her arm was totally inconsistent with total paralysis. She also complained of profound weakness in her left leg, but in its resting position, the position of the leg did not indicate any significant weakness. As I talked to her, I recognized something in her demeanor that I had seen before. I find it hard to describe what that means, but suffice to say, this recognition is an art one learns over the years and is honed with experience. Unfortunately, this art is fast disappearing. As a result, an enormous amount of money is spent on doing multiple tests and repeating them because a patient's condition is either unchanged or getting worse. Besides the financial costs, which are huge, patients' continued suffering is even more costly. It not only disrupts their own lives, it also creates a ripple effect throughout their families and their communities.

The magnitude of this medical problem is immense. Psychosomatic illness is a worldwide phenomenon, according to a study conducted by the World Health Organization in 1997. This finding still holds true today. Twenty percent of those who saw their doctors were shown to have psychosomatic disorders. Further studies support this finding. Ten to 20 percent of all patients seen by primary-care physicians meet the criteria for psychosomatic disorders. (RL Spitzer. 1994. JAMA; K. Kroenke. 2002. *Psychosomatic Medicine*; Br J de Waal MW. 2004. *Psychiatry*; I.A. Arnold. 2009. *Psychosomatics*). This is not always immediately obvious because stress also manifests itself in actual conditions, such as chronic headaches, insomnia, and depression, which are not psychosomatic.

Freeing Patients from the Tyranny of their Minds

To successfully treat a psychosomatic ailment, physicians must recognize that the patient has become a victim of her own mind. In this state, she is not only vulnerable to additional stress, she is also highly suggestible. If a doctor diagnoses a serious illness, the patient will believe she has it. On the other hand, if a doctor tells the patient she is getting better, she will believe that, too. That's why it is so important to be positive when you are dealing with a psychosomatic illness.

Survival is a basic human drive. At a subconscious level, patients want to get better; they simply do not know how to break through the mental block that is holding them back. I told Hilda I could help diffuse this block. I used a benign, non-threatening technique—massaging her neck—while at the same time, assuring her that she was indeed improving. She believed me. First, she started to move her fingers, then, her hand, and finally, she was able to lift her entire arm. The strength in her arm and leg returned to normal in less than five minutes, and she could walk without any assistance. This was not a miracle; it was good, old-fashioned medicine—observing the patient, listening to her, understanding what was causing her stress, and reading the MRI.

Even as I was able help Hilda at that moment, I knew the relapse rate in such circumstances is high. I would have to investigate and treat the stress factors contributing to her "paralysis." This can only happen in a healthy physician-patient relationship. Such relationships have been the bedrock of medical care for centuries, but they are rapidly being eroded since the introduction of EHR.

The important question is why wasn't Hilda's condition picked up before she received tPA, a drug with potentially dangerous outcomes? I found the answers when I reviewed her voluminous physician-generated EHRs. Each of the doctors had spent much more time on the computer, recording her entire clinical history and examination, than they had spent with Hilda. Considering how busy they are in ER, doctors barely have enough time to spend with patients as it is; if they are required to record every detail of the visit in the patient's EHR, patient-doctor time is reduced even further. There is no time to ask them about any stress in their lives or about their family situations.

Hilda told me that her younger sister had recently suffered a stroke, causing her to be paralyzed on the left side, and Hilda had assumed the role of caregiver. Was this history relevant? Absolutely, if I wanted to treat Hilda and heal the root cause of her problem.

This art of practicing medicine takes many years to learn, and going beyond the obvious symptoms by asking simple questions is part of that art. I pride myself in taking the necessary time to listen to and examine my patients, but, frankly, the pressure of trying to complete the EHR in the allotted time is getting to me. I find myself just focusing on all the symptoms that have been recorded in the records, just as Hilda's doctors did, without really asking questions. Had the ER doctors actually spent some time with Hilda, I am certain they would have discovered her real problem.

Over a hundred years ago, Sir William Osler, who helped usher in modern medicine, said, "Medicine is learned by the bedside and not in the classroom. Let not your conceptions of disease come from words heard in the lecture room or read from the book. See, and then reason and compare and control. But see first." These words are still worth heeding.

The Mental and Physical Consequences of Stress

Recent scientific evidence explains how the mind affects organic functions and what happens to one's body may be linked to emotional stress. Changes do occur due to stress— some rapidly and others over time—in the immune, cardiovascular, hormonal, and autonomic systems, which in turn, can affect the functioning of the nervous system. In his classic book, *Anatomy of an Illness as Perceived by the Patient*, Norman Cousins observed the importance of this phenomenon: "The greatest force in the human body is the natural drive of the body to heal itself, but that force is not independent of the belief system. Everything begins with a belief." Did

Hilda perceive an illness in her mind, which then appeared in her body?

I still love watching the video we made that documents Hilda's remarkable recovery. I show it to other physicians and medical staff in training to emphasize the importance of listening to and observing a patient and only then performing a good clinical examination to arrive at a diagnosis. Today, unfortunately, a computer in the examination room commands more of the doctor's attention than the patient does. The patient's complaints have been entered into the EHR by a nurse; further examination and tests are based on those records.

It is like an assembly line in a factory, with one patient following another within a predetermined timeframe. Increasingly, no emotions are expressed or shared, and the doctor hardly connects with the patient. I would have totally missed Hilda's condition if I had brought a computer into the room. Without one, I had the time to observe her closely and hear what she was saying. The clinical diagnostic tools I had learned during my training helped me arrive at a correct diagnosis, which in turn led to her remarkable recovery.

Now, one would think that a doctor would conduct an independent evaluation of a patient the first time he sees her. That used to be the norm, but with the change in regulations and mandatory EHR, procedures have changed. Because doctors have so little unrushed time to spend with patients, they have been forced to narrow their focus to just one symptom, rather than trying to discover what is really going on. Sadly, most physicians have given up fighting the system. They no longer practice medicine as they did in the past; they are now constrained by directives established by nonmedical administrators. In his online newsletter, *The Doctor Weighs*

In, Kevin Campbell, MD, an internationally recognized cardiologist, wrote the following: "Physicians have become worker bees in the factory of the administrative overlords."

EHR: A Blessing or a Curse?

It is extremely difficult to change a diagnosis once it is incorrectly entered into the EHR. Recently, I was visiting a clinic in Blaine, Michigan, to give a talk to a number of physicians and mid-level practitioners. Just before my talk, I casually asked them about their experience with EHR. One of the senior nurse practitioners of twenty-eight years, Ann Rechtzigel, quickly pointed out that EHR is the "next best thing since sliced bread." She explained how it has become so much easier to retrieve medical data on a patient who may have been seen at some of their other clinic locations. In the past, she would have to wait to receive such data. Now, it is all on the computer, easily accessible. Some of the younger physicians echoed her feelings and indicated how pleased they are with EHR. They would not want to go back to paper charts.

I mentioned to them how patient-doctor, face-to-face time is significantly reduced with EHR, and as a result, we may not be effectively connecting with our patients. Since medicine is all about observation and listening, the diagnosis we arrive at may not always be accurate. They were all in total agreement with what I said and, in fact, mentioned a few studies that proved my point. They liked EHR because of its logistical advantage of retrieving data but were quick to point out that "caring" for patients is, in fact, compromised. And, yet, they all favored EHR. They appeared to be more focused on the mechanics than on truly caring for the patients.

It is frightening because this problem of "mechanics over caring" is readily accepted by medical students and residents in training, and if this not corrected, we will undo the hard-won progress made over the years. For the younger generation, reliance on digital technologies is not only attractive but addictive. One of my nurses complained of how her teenage daughter texted her from her bedroom to inquire when dinner would be ready! The breakroom at many clinics where staff once used to talk and share their stories has become very quiet because people are focused on their smart phones. Many studies have concluded that this behavior adversely affects communication skills over time.

In hospital- or clinic-driven surveys designed to capture patient satisfaction, the major complaint is that patients spend very little time with their doctors. It takes time for a personal bond to develop between a doctor and a patient, but the current system severely curtails the time allowed for an office visit. There is a growing concern in the medical community about the regulations being imposed by Congress and other federal agencies, which put financial gains before patient care. The people who passed these laws and regulations may not be standing in our exam rooms, but their influence is palpable. Politicians tell physicians what software to use in their offices, which EHR options must be employed during an office visit, and how they will be penalized if they do not follow mandated guidelines. The noose physicians feel is already around their necks is being slowly tightened and will eventually choke the life out of the patient-physician relationship.

Having to deal with digital technology related to EHR is no different. In fact, it is even worse, since here we are dealing directly with human lives where lack of proper communication can have serious consequences. I was recently talking to a young physician who had been using EHR for the past two years. He shared a very interesting story with me.

It was a busy day in the clinic, and as was his habit, he opened up the patient's electronic chart to review it before going into the examination room to see her. He reviewed her last clinic visit notes, her current medications, and her most recent laboratory results, which revealed that her blood glucose was running high. He looked at the patient's current complaints of pains in her feet, which were well summarized by the nurse. He ordered a nerve conduction study to make sure the patient did not have a condition called neuropathy due to her diabetes. Then, he electronically prescribed an oral medicine for her leg discomfort and adjusted her diabetic medications on her electronic med-sheet.

When he finished with that chart, he opened the one belonging to the next patient. An hour later, the patient with diabetes went to the nursing desk to ask why the doctor had not come to see her. It was only then that the young doctor realized he had totally forgotten to see the patient! He had, in fact, treated the "iPatient,"—the virtual patient, connected to the EHR— instead of the "real" patient. This is one of the dangers of interacting with the computer rather than the human being.

The Power of a Healthy Doctor-Patient Relationship

There are many more patients like Hilda whose diagnoses can only be made by observing and listening. Tests alone will not diagnose their illnesses. Once the diagnosis is made, the doctor-patient relationship is a cornerstone of a positive therapeutic outcome for patients. Knowing your patients, knowing their families, and knowing what they struggle with, day in and day out, are the elements that lead to healthy doctor-patient relationships. A physician dispenses a lot more than a prescription. A physician's attitude also becomes a part of the therapy.

Several scientific studies support the significant therapeutic value of a healthy relationship between doctor and patient. In a controlled study of a placebo versus a real antidepressant drug in depressed patients, a good relationship turned out to be more powerful in promoting recovery from depression than whether the patient had received an active treatment or the placebo.

Especially powerful is the connection the patient feels with her doctor. Does she like him, trust him, respect him? This connection is a powerful healing energy. If doctors are no longer able to share this energy with their patients, billions of dollars will be lost because it will take patients a very long time to recover, if they recover at all. Most importantly, the quality of care suffers. The main objective of EHR is to improve quality of care, not to erode it.

EHR, however, is a boon for hospitals. AMA president, Dr. Steven J. Stack, said it so well: "EHRs have been essentially reduced to a tool for billing." In a fee-for-service payment system, EHR makes sure that no procedures are overlooked. Every encounter, every procedure is now captured and billed. Cutting, pasting, and importing already populated information on multiple medical issues the patient may now have, or has ever had, goes into the records. Every click of a button allows for higher billing for a physician without improving quality of care to patients.

Before EHR, hospital administrators constantly reminded doctors to record as many medical conditions as possible to improve reimbursement. Recently, while looking up EHR for laboratory results I had ordered for a patient hospitalized for fewer than forty-eight hours, I counted at least thirty blood-glucose reports (finger-stick tests that diabetic patients routinely do on their own at home but are now performed by nurses at the hospital). Undoubtedly, these were captured by the sophisticated billing programs attached to EHR. Adapting to EHR has allowed hospitals to let go of many personnel, while refusing to hire data-entry employees (citing cost as a reason), which would free up doctors from this task and allow them to spend more in-person time with their patients.

The Myth of EHR "Confidentiality"

I was also not aware of this interesting fact: EHRs of patients are purchased by pharmaceutical companies for a hefty price. The hospitals do not inform patients of this. EHRs are made available to state health agencies, which in turn sell the information to interested parties. Even though the names and addresses are redacted, the records do contain a lot of other information, such as the patients' age, detailed medical history, when they were seen by doctors, and when they were hospitalized—all of which makes patients vulnerable to identification.

In an article by Jordan Robertson in *Bloomberg Businessweek* (August 2013), Latanya Sweeney, director of Harvard University's Data Privacy Lab, identified thirty-five patients from a Washington state database by buying state medical data and creating a simple software program to cross-reference that information with news reports and other public records. "All I have to know is a little bit about patients and when they went to a hospital, and I can find their identity."

Robertson goes on to say that this data-mining industry, which buys the information and resells it to medical companies, will top $10 billion in revenue by 2020.

My medical colleagues with whom I shared this information were shocked to know that their patients' EHRs were traded for money! Do patients know this? Should they be properly informed about this, as well as the fact that they could be identified by insurance companies to raise their premiums? It is no secret that some of the bigger health-insurance companies are spending increasing amounts of money to purchase patients' EHRs. Robertson quotes Jim Pyles, a principal at Powers Pyles Sutter & Verville law firm, which specializes in health law and policy: "In an era of increasingly sophisticated hacking, electronic health information is like nuclear energy. If it's harnessed and kept under tight control, it has potential for good. But if it gets out of control, the damage is incalculable."

In 2015, 78.8 million Anthem Insurance customers were hacked. It was the largest healthcare breach ever. More than 113 million medical records were compromised in 2016, according to the Office of Civil Rights (OCR) under Health and Human Services. Cyber-hacking of EHRs ranked second in US data breaches in 2015 and placed in the top ten on Verizon's global hacking report. This will only get worse because "Electronic health records are one hundred times more valuable than stolen credit cards," says James Scott, co-founder and senior fellow at the Institute for Critical Infrastructure Technology (ICIT) in Washington, D.C. "A single Medicare or Medicaid electronic health record can fetch $500," according to Scott.

The cost of EHR is quite prohibitive for solo practitioners. Several studies estimate the cost of owning and installing

EHR ranges from $15,000 to $70,000 per provider. This cost is just the tip of the iceberg. Many studies now confirm that clinics are seeing fewer patients per day since acquiring EHR. Doctors are spending more time "typing" and maneuvering their way through the program. The extra time they allocate for each patient visit does not translate into more informal time with that patient. On the contrary, that time is significantly shortened.

While the patient is in front of you, and you want to check the laboratory results, it takes three clicks to get there; for MRI results, it takes three additional clicks; to review meds, it takes three additional clicks. Once you have closed the "chart," if the patient has forgotten to ask you for a prescription refill, it takes many more clicks to send the prescription to the patient's pharmacy. It is also important to enter the prescription correctly, or it will not reach the pharmacy.

I did a small experiment in our own clinic. I acted as a patient and then asked one of our "super and advanced EPIC users" (those who train doctors to use this software) some of the usual questions patients would normally ask during their routine visit. After I posed the question, I looked up the answer in the paper chart, while she looked it up in the EHR. I had the results nine minutes faster than my advanced EPIC user!

Not only did I have the results faster, but I was able to look at her during the extra time I saved. I never seemed to be disconnected from her, while she hardly looked at me because she was busy clicking away on the computer. Even when she read the reports of various tests I requested, she could not take her gaze off the computer screen. She talked to me, but the computer demanded her focus. This is what is really driving the majority of the physicians insane. They complain, they protest, but no one listens to them. What's worse is that, if they do not comply, they are chastised and have their year-end bonuses—a substantial part of their of income—reduced.

The Most Common Cause of Physician Burnout

Physicians are caught between a rock and a hard place. Like a pressure cooker, the frustration piles up until they cannot handle any more. The end result is that the physicians either give up being "physicians to their patients," or they burn out. In a 2016 study published in *Mayo Clinic Proceedings*, mandatory use of electronic health records was identified as the most common cause of physician burnout.

Researchers at the Mayo Clinic looked at several months of 2014 survey data from 6,560 US physicians, which measured features of work life, including burnout, and entered data into a computer. Even after controlling for such factors as age, sex, specialty, and the number of hours doctors work per week, the researchers found a strong link between burnout and time spent doing digital work. Of the many physicians who used EHR, 44 percent were dissatisfied, and nearly 63 percent of doctors believed that EHR made their jobs less efficient. Nearly half said that they spent an unreasonable amount of time on clerical tasks related to patient care. "The clerical burden associated with electronic health records has been a major contributing factor to physician burnout, with computerized physician order entry as the biggest source of frustration," says Dr. Tait Shanafelt, the lead author of a study on the issue and director of the Mayo Clinic Department of Medicine Program on Physician Well-Being.

There are aspects of an EHR that are clearly useful, e.g., patient demographic information, medical history including health insurance information, whom to contact in an emergency, etc. It is much more convenient to have this information in an electronic database.

However, just as they have messed up the rest of the healthcare delivery and financing system, government bureaucrats and overzealous hospital administrators have taken what is a good idea and bungled it. They have dumped all the clerical stuff on physicians and nurses, which takes their valuable time away from patents.

Some physicians, who are financially able to, employ scribes to do all their data entry. Their experience is unanimously positive. It allows them to spend more time with their patients, and in fact, some report that they can see a couple of more patients in a day than they used to. However, the hospital or clinic administrators do not care to undertake this extra cost.

And contrary to the common myth, studies have shown that physicians—especially older ones—are not technophobes or dinosaurs. They adapt to technology very quickly and readily if it improves patient care. When the technology is right and the need is there, an appropriate digital device will be invented to foster and preserve the physician-patient relationship.

Some of the younger physicians in training in my department once remarked that I "hated" EHR because I was from the older, non-digital generation. I did not agree with them, and to prove my point, I did a small experiment. I asked three of the younger doctors, who "loved" EHR, to each see the same patient, to take full history, and to examine the patient. They were to do this separately, one at a time. First, I asked them to do it the old-fashioned way, without any computer in the room. For a second patient, I asked them to take the computer with them into the room and to do it the "new way." After they were done, I asked them a simple question, "Can you write down for me on a piece of paper the color of your patient's eyes?" They were 100 percent correct when they had each examined the patient the "old-fashioned" way and completely wrong when they brought a computer into the room. If they missed such an important clinical observation while they were engaged with a computer, rather than the patient, how could they arrive at a correct diagnosis?

Today's medical students will care for tomorrow's patients. To ensure and preserve the medical excellence for which this country has been recognized, progress needs to continue, and, inevitably, changes will be made. But they should not be made at the expense of what we have already achieved and learned over the years. The consequences of this loss would be catastrophic. The pain inflicted on physicians by mandatory use of EHR is literally killing them, exacerbating the current healthcare crisis. One way to avoid this crisis is to find another way to handle the clerical aspect of EHR; in other words, remove it from the physicians' list of responsibilities. This one action would improve physicians' ability to function more effectively.

Chapter 3
Physicians in Harm's Way: Turning Medical Practices into War Zones

"Burnout at its deepest level is not the result of some train wreck of examinations, long call shifts, or poor clinical evaluations. It is the sum total of hundreds and thousands of tiny betrayals of purpose, each one so minute that it hardly attracts notice. When a great ship steams across the ocean, even tiny ripples can accumulate over time, precipitating a dramatic shift in course."
—Richard Gunderman, MD
Chancellor's Professor, Schools of Medicine, Liberal Arts, and Philanthropy
Indiana University, Indianapolis, IN

First, there was a loud, deafening noise. Then, the skies turned dirty with sand and smoke, just a couple of miles from where he was. As he rushed out toward the tent that housed the Forward Resuscitative Surgery System (FRSS), hot sand from the blast hit his face like hundreds of tiny needles.

Dr. P was less than a mile away from the combat zone in Iraq. Just the day before, he and nine others from his team had set up the mobile trauma unit, generators, lighting, equipment, and all the medical and surgical supplies in a record thirty minutes to provide immediate emergency care to injured soldiers within a mile of active fighting.

* * * * *

Medical corpsmen provide on-the-spot first-aid as wounded soldiers are rushed to FRSS, where a second level of care is provided. This unit is equipped to handle up to sixteen trauma surgeries before needing to be re-supplied.

Once stabilized, patients are quickly moved to level 3 care in Baghdad or Ballad, which offers the highest level of medical care available within the combat zone. Then, they are moved to level 4 in Landstuhl, Germany, where they are given medical and surgical care outside the combat zone; and, finally, they are transported to level 5 in Bethesda, Maryland. This level of care is specifically designed to provide soldiers with maximum return to function through a combination of medical, surgical, rehabilitative, and convalescent care.

Operating in the Thick of Battle

Dr. P, a trauma surgeon in the mobile FRSS unit, was trained to perform major surgeries under the most horrifying conditions, but never did he imagine he would be operating continuously for ten hours a day in a tent as big as an average American living room. Temperatures inside the tent often rose up to 110 degrees Fahrenheit, flies swarmed over the bodies of the soldiers, and mortars exploded nearby as Dr. P explored the twenty-five feet of a soldier's intestines, inch by inch, trying to find tears caused by an explosion that had ripped into the man's abdomen.

The first hour following injury is absolutely critical to treatment and survival. Units like Dr. P's have revolutionized the way critically injured soldiers are now being treated. By reducing the time of receiving vital care to their wounds, the chances of surviving injuries have increased significantly.

Dr. P was deployed to Iraq's Al Anbar Province in 2006, when armed conflict against the American-led military coalition had markedly escalated. He was on call around the clock and in a constant state of readiness. Dr. P shared the following with me:

"You never really know when casualties are going to come in. I can usually tell by the intensity of explosions and by the huge clouds forming in the sky that it is going to be a bad, nasty day. There are days when I hardly get any sleep or any time to eat; but when I see a wounded soldier brought in, struggling for his life, nothing matters more to me than to resuscitate and stabilize him until he is safely transferred to a medical facility, away from the active fighting zone.

"Sometimes, the wounded men are too weak to speak, but a gentle touch of their hands on mine to convey their thanks means everything to me. This is the moment every physician hopes to experience, to remind him of why he embarked on the long, arduous journey of becoming a doctor.

"That simple touch is so powerful that it takes away all my pains and rejuvenates me enough to move on to my next patient. It's a feeling no one can ever explain. Sometimes, their eyes speak to me because they are too weak to even move their hands. No matter what we do for them, it is never thankless."

* * * * *

Now, within minutes of Dr. P's reaching the surgical tent, the first casualty arrives. He takes a quick look at the young soldier and immediately requests that an urgent page be sent out for blood. The soldier was bleeding profusely, everywhere. His abdomen is torn open, his spleen is like pulp, his liver is damaged, one kidney is crushed, and part of his face is torn apart. He is gasping for air and, unless Dr. P can get a tube down his throat and into his trachea through which air can be pumped in and out, he will quickly die.

As the nurse anesthetist secures the man's airway, Dr. P stops the hemorrhaging from the soldier's main arteries by placing a tourniquet around his left upper arm near his shoulder and around his left thigh, just below the groin. Now Dr. P has to do something very quickly to stop the bleeding from the soldier's torso.

One of the corpsmen is already infusing a 5 percent albumin (protein solution) into the soldier as quickly as possible. Several soldiers with the same blood type have already arrived at the tent. One of the nurses starts to collect their blood and, within fifteen minutes of his arrival, the soldier is rapidly receiving life-saving, warm blood.

The Walking Blood Bank

Other soldiers take turns donating their blood and wait near the tent until blood is no longer required. This "walking blood bank" is the lifeline for many soldiers who, otherwise, would die due to excessive blood loss. All soldiers know their blood type and, as soon as a page goes out for a particular type, soldiers report immediately to the trauma unit.

The wounded soldier was unconscious and in shock when he arrived, but now, his caregivers can feel his pulse faintly at his wrist and, even though his blood pressure is still very low, he is being prepped for surgery to stop the bleeding from his abdomen.

Dr. P's main focus is to save the soldier, to keep him alive. Dr. P first removes the spleen, then the crushed kidney, and, finally, a part of the soldier's torn liver. The bleeding from the soldier's torso has stopped. His blood pressure has risen, while warm blood was still being infused into him continuously.

Three hours have elapsed. Dr. P has to do something quickly to restore blood supply to the soldier's extremities. Otherwise, he will be forced to amputate the soldier's arm at his shoulder and the leg at his groin.

Dr. P recently completed training on inserting temporary Argyle shunts to connect two ends of torn arteries and allow blood to flow distally. The most tedious part of this surgery is finding and securing the two ends of a torn artery because blood vessels retract after they are severed. He had never placed such a shunt in a live patient before, nor had he ever done such major abdominal surgery on someone for whom every second was critical to survival.

First, he removes the tourniquet from the soldier's arm; blood gushes out of the man's axillary artery, flooding the field of surgery. With the help of an aide who gently compresses the soldier's arm proximally, the field of surgery becomes a little clearer. Dr. P is now able to dissect, explore, and finally locate the proximal end of the torn artery. He puts a clamp on it and then starts to look for the distal end of the artery. This proves to be a challenging task. If he doesn't find it in another ten minutes, he will have to abort the procedure and sacrifice the arm in favor of the leg.

Finally, Dr. P finds the other end, instructs the nurse to push heparin solution into both ends of the blood vessel to flush out any clots, and then secures the two ends with an Argyle shunt. He opens the clamps to let blood flow once again into an arm that was almost dead.

He then turns to the leg. This is a somewhat easier task, because the artery in the leg is of a larger caliber. Dr. P is able to find the two ends and connect them via a shunt. Blood begins to flow into the soldier's leg, but his blood pressure is dropping. Dr. P has to give him more blood.

The nurse inserts another intravenous line, and the limbs start to warm up. Within ten minutes, the aide reports that a pulse can be felt distally in both limbs!

The soldier's intestines are next. Some parts of the man's gut had been ruptured, so Dr. P dissects out the damaged section of intestine and carefully connects its two ends. Satisfied that there are no more tears in the remaining twenty feet of intestine, Dr. P thoroughly cleans the soldier's abdomen with normal saline and sutures up the abdominal wall.

Six hours have passed since Dr. P started operating on this soldier. He then turns to other casualties that need his attention. Fortunately, there are not any life-threatening injuries. Dr. P approaches a twenty-five-year-old soldier whose leg is completely crushed; it is not salvageable. The soldier is already prepped and ready for Dr. P to amputate his leg just below the groin.

After this procedure, Dr. P examines other casualties with large, gaping wounds, which he cleans and sutures. By this time, he has been operating for ten hours.

Exhausted but Elated

Wearily, he returns to the recovery tent to check on his first patient. To his delight, that soldier is waking up and moving all his extremities to commands. The nurse reports that he has received a total of fifty units of blood. Dr. P kneels down and lifts the urine bag that is hanging below the soldier's cot. Seeing that it is about half full brings a huge smile to Dr. P's face.

Urine output is a very good indicator of effective fluid resuscitation. If the therapy is not effective, urine output drops dramatically.

Dr. P's tiredness is gone, and he feels elated. Never before has he gotten so much joy and satisfaction at seeing half a liter of urine!

"This soldier will live with all four of his limbs! He should be stable enough to be transferred to Ballad for further care in the morning," Dr. P says out loud.

He is overjoyed with the results of Argyle shunts and, in the ensuing months, he would use them at least twenty-five times with a 95.5 percent success rate! This means that twenty-four of twenty-five soldiers would not lose their limbs, a remarkable outcome that would be reported in a medical journal in the months to come.

Even though all soldiers wear protective armor, they are vulnerable in their axillary and groin areas. These areas have no protection to allow for mobility. Insurgents know this and, therefore, specifically target these areas. Injuries in these regions cause severe and fatal bleeding due to the rupture of axillary or femoral arteries—unless, of course, a tourniquet is applied to save the patient. In turn, tourniquets can cause irreparable ischemic destruction of the limb, which has to be sacrificed unless the tourniquet can be removed within six hours.

Penetrating injuries to the extremities account for up to 75 percent of wounds sustained during combat. Hemorrhage is the leading cause of preventable death. The age-old saying "saving a life for a limb" is no longer acceptable, thanks to FRSS and its use of temporary vascular shunting.

Filled with relief, Dr. P sits down to write brief notes on each of the patients he had treated that day. He describes what the problem was, what had been done, and what actions are still needed. Then, he pins the notes to the chests of those soldiers to inform the doctors who would be receiving the wounded in the morning.

"This works very well—better than having to enter all this information into a computer. Doing that takes up a lot of my time and pulls me away from saving lives. I have never received any complaints from doctors. In fact, they like it because it saves them time, inasmuch as they find these notes to be precise and to the point!" Dr. P explains.

After finishing his medical records, Dr. P retires to his tent for some sleep, knowing full well he will be awakened several times during the night to respond to emergent medical issues on patients he has operated on. And yes, it will be a repeat of the day if more casualties arrive from renewed fighting.

What is Waiting at Home

Dr. P's one-year deployment was now coming to an end. He had operated daily for twelve months, seven days a week, putting in some one hundred hours a week, and working under the harshest imaginable conditions. He had survived mortars which, quite often, would land just outside his tent. He had operated when temperatures in the tent were unbearable. For that long year, he had been under a constant state of emergency and readiness to report to the operating room even when he had had very little sleep. He was now ready to return home to his family. The offer he had received—to join a growing multispecialty practice as a trauma surgeon in a large metropolitan city in the United States—was very appealing.

"Hey, they want you to do twenty-four-hour shifts only eight days a month! Pay is not the greatest, but they promise you a handsome year-end bonus. Go for it!" advised an orthopedic friend who had just joined Dr. P's FRSS unit.

Dr. P signed the contract. Getting a lawyer to review the document never crossed his mind. The important aspects of his employment were very clear and easy to understand. He would be paid for working 192 hours a month; the rest of the time was his to enjoy as he wished. A non-compete clause—not to practice within a twenty-mile radius from their place of practice for a year after leaving that practice—was standard. He was eager and ready to start. Having served his country while in harm's way for a year would make the rest of his career as a physician in the States seem like a piece of cake—or so he thought.

Culture Shock

Now, eight years into that state-side job, Dr. P feels defeated as a physician. "The practice of medicine has become a business. I feel trapped in this corporate world of medicine," he says. "Life is being sucked out of me. I can't breathe freely."

During a twenty-four-hour shift, Dr. P sees more than fifty patients. Some require urgent surgeries for trauma (mostly auto accidents and gunshot wounds), which take most of his time. Then, he has to "round" on an entire fifteen-bed trauma ICU and look in on a similar number of patients on a regular floor. In between, he takes calls from eleven other hospitals related to the transfer of patients with major trauma. He doesn't mind doing all this work. In fact, he feels best when he is with patients and treating them.

What is killing him is the administrative work he is required to do. For every patient he sees, for every phone call he makes, he has to record everything in great detail, electronically. He is required to type all of his notes in his patients' EHRs. He has to list every symptom, whether or not the patient smokes, detailed family and medication histories, general and specific system examinations, everything he said to the patient and what he did for the patient, all tests he ordered, and medications he prescribed.

All of this must be done electronically so that the clinic can easily bill insurance companies to the fullest. Now, one would think that, as physicians, we should be doing all of this anyway. The problem is that doing it this way takes a lot of time. What a far cry from the way Dr. P was used to keeping records in the FRSS unit!

Recent studies have shown that for every hour of time spent with a patient, a physician puts in two hours doing administrative work. As a result, doctors like Dr. P., who are contracted to do only twenty-four-hour shifts, eight days a month, end up being at the hospital every day to do administrative work, sometimes putting in more than eight hours a day on that alone.

Lately, Dr. P has been working from home as well. The sad part is that he does not get reimbursed for any of the extra time he puts in. If he doesn't do his charting electronically, the records will show him to be "delinquent." If his administrative work is not completed in a timely fashion, his year-end bonus could be adversely impacted, or, worse yet, he could be fired from his job.

There has been a steady increase in the number of patients physicians care for, approximately by 25 percent each year. Yet, instead of seeing an increase in take-home pay, doctors' salaries have declined. Bonuses have been slashed drastically. A plea to get a secretary or an additional mid-level healthcare provider to help ease this burden is always met with the same answer from administrators: "We don't have the budget for that." In contrast, the number of administrators is increasing at a rapid rate, and they are being paid more each year.

As a result of all this extra work, Dr. P has very little time to exercise. He has cut down on social activities in favor of spending more time with his family.

"I dread going to work," he admits. "I have become a factory worker. Everything I endured while serving my country in the FRSS unit pales before all the bullshit I have to put up with. Sadly, hardly any of what I do is directly related to the actual care of my patients. Caring for patients while my life was in constant danger in Iraq didn't do it, but administrators have succeeded in breaking me! My other colleagues, who never served in the armed forces, feel the same way. We all want to leave, but the question is—where do we go? This problem is not unique to us. It is going on throughout the country, and it's getting worse. Besides, uprooting our families is not an easy task."

When I asked Dr. P if he and his other colleagues in the department ever supported each other by talking about these problems, his answer was unnerving. "We all talk about our problems, and then we get even more depressed. No one has anything positive to say or can offer a solution to the problem."

Suffering in Silence

Dr. P doesn't discuss his feelings with anyone else, either—not even his wife—because, as he puts it, "What can they do? We need a major shake-up in the medical community, an uprising, a revolution, to stop and reverse the atrocities being systematically laid upon physicians."

Another issue that tore him apart was an allegation by one of his patients that Dr. P had neglected to care for him appropriately. A lawsuit ensued and, even though the jury clearly sided with the doctor, this experience left him terrified. He is constantly reminded of it and, as a result, has been ordering more tests for his patients "just to make sure." In addition, he spends extra time documenting in great detail everything he does.

According to a study published in the *Journal of the American College of Surgeons* in November 2011, by Charles M. Balch, MD, PhD, FACS, a professor of surgery at the University of Texas Southwestern Medical Center in Dallas, "Malpractice lawsuits can take a profound personal toll on surgeons and can cause psychological distress and career burnout." This experience has definitely had profoundly negative effects on Dr. P.

As he explained to me, "This is so much worse than being in the war zone! We do not deliberately want to harm patients. No physician would ever want to do that. Even if you are found not negligent, there are serious negative repercussions for being sued. It makes you feel worthless, and you become very defensive in all that you do. The soldiers I cared for appreciated what I did for them, and even the higher-ups in command sincerely acknowledged all the sacrifices we made."

Dr. P recalled an event from his time in Iraq. Several units and their commanders had gathered to pay a tribute to one of their fallen soldiers. Insurgents found out and ambushed the gathering, causing severe injuries to at least forty soldiers. Dr. P and his team sprang into action and worked non-stop for twenty-two hours, saving all of them. The following day, a chief surgeon flew in from Baghdad to personally thank Dr. P's team. "He was one of those stern, rigid, macho Army guys who never show their emotions. But as he gave a brief speech, he choked up, and tears rolled down his cheeks. However, he quickly controlled himself, looked into my eyes, shook my hand, and left. That look in his eyes said it all! I have never felt as appreciated in my entire life as I did at that moment. And he didn't even say a word to me directly or pat me on my back. It was all in his eyes.

"In contrast, the administrators in my clinic here want more and more from us, always finding ways to increase our work load, without any additional financial compensation. We are asked to actively take part in various committees and attend meetings. These meetings have nothing to do with improving the care of patients or the status of physicians. Administrators are geared toward improving their image, attracting more business, and bolstering their interests."

Dr. P continued. "Granted, that participation is all on a 'volunteer basis,' but not attending the meetings would be seriously considered when handing out year-end bonuses. I feel like being a cog in this ever-revolving wheel. I hope there is a change, soon, before it's too late."

Most of the problems for physicians intensified with the enactment of the ACA in March 2010. The Trump administration and the Republican Congress tried and failed to repeal and replace the ACA but ignored any changes to the parts of the law that favor corporate ownership of private practices, even though it is physicians and not large corporate entities who are best equipped to care for patients.

Dr. P envies those who say they love their jobs and look forward to going to work each day. When I asked why he was unhappy, even though he works fewer hours now than he did while in the armed forces, Dr. P said, "The one year I spent in the FRSS unit was the best year in my career as a physician. If it weren't for my family, I would go back in a heartbeat— away from this craziness that is destroying the art of true healing. More than half of what I am forced to do now has nothing to with healing the patient. Being in the active fighting zone is regarded as being 'in harm's way,' but, for me, it is just the opposite. Being a physician now in the States is truly what I would regard as being in harm's way!"

Chapter 4

ICD-10 Codes: Helping or Hindering Quality of Care?

"If freedom of speech is taken away, then dumb and silent
we may be led, like sheep to the slaughter."
—George Washington (1783)

T risha knew, at age six, that she wanted to be a doctor. After twelve years in elementary, middle, and high school; four years of undergraduate work at a university; four more years of medical school; and yet another four years in a residency program, she began work as a family-practice physician in a large medical group. By then, she was thirty-two years old. The friends with whom she had grown up were already married, had children, and were well settled. However, to Trisha, her career was worth the sacrifices she had made to become a doctor. She was happiest when she was caring for patients but far less happy when she found herself fighting with insurance companies on behalf of her patients, entering hundreds of details into a computer, and trying not to run afoul of the latest policies and procedures put in place by her employer.

The situation became even worse in 2014 when a large health-insurance company bought the clinic in which she was working and instituted new procedures. Trisha was now expected to see up to twenty-four patients a day. A follow-up patient was scheduled every fifteen minutes, a new patient

65

every thirty minutes. The insurance company directed the clinic staff to first schedule patients with Medicare Advantage Capitated Plans—HMO or PPC plans that allow payment of a flat fee for each covered patient—and to record as many medical issues as possible. The more medical issues recorded, the greater the capitated income *per* patient *per* year. A capitated payment arrangement is when a set amount is paid to healthcare providers for each patient assigned to them during a certain period of time.

ICD-10 Coding—"A catastrophic disruption"

In October 2015, the Centers for Medicare & Medicaid Services (CMS) made it mandatory to use International Classification of Diseases, Tenth Revision (ICD-10) codes to report all diagnoses with associated complications. ICD-10 had expanded the 13,000 codes in ICD-9, which Trisha had been using, to 164,000 codes, allowing a greater degree of specific clinical information to be entered. The transition required a great deal of advanced planning and preparation. Not only was new software installed and tested but medical practices had to provide training for physicians, staff members, and administrators. Along with these changes, it was necessary to draft new policies and guidelines, as well as update paperwork and forms. Medical practitioners who created "crosswalks" to convert their most frequently used ICD-9-CM (Clinical Modification) codes to the ICD-10-CM equivalents were required to attend several training classes to learn the system.

The AMA had long opposed implementation of ICD-10 codes. AMA President Robert Wah, MD, correctly predicted "a catastrophic disruption to physician practices with implementation of these codes." In an address to the AMA's House of Delegates in November 2014, Dr. Wah characterized the planned implementation of ICD-10 as similar to the dark forces that controlled the galaxy in *Star Wars*. He noted that "... each of the six *Star Wars* films had this line: *I have a bad feeling about this.*"

Anne Zieger reported in *Health Care DIVE* (June 2014) that Dr. Wah wasn't even sure ICD-10 would improve patient care. A survey by the American Health Information Management Association and the eHealth Initiatives found that 38 percent of providers thought revenue would decrease in the year following a switch from ICD-9 to ICD-10, while only 6 percent thought revenue would increase.

A broad-based healthcare industry advocacy group—consisting of big insurance companies, such as the BlueCross BlueShield Association, America's Health Insurance Plans, and the Advanced Medical Technology Association—reacted fiercely to Dr. Wah's criticism of ICD-10, saying: "It is hard to fathom why anyone would promote having our national data fail to meet the demands of twenty-first century healthcare. How can we as a nation assess hospital outcomes, pay fairly, ensure accurate performance reports, and embrace value-based care if our coded data doesn't provide such basic information?" The group, which had a vested interest in the outcome of this debate, asked, "Doesn't the public have a right to know this kind of information?"

An excellent report, "Disease Classification (ICD-10): Doctors and Patients Will Pay," published in *Healthcare Reform* by the Heritage Foundation, was presented by John Grimsley and John S. O'Shea, MD. Grimsley is a graduate fellow at the Center for Health Policy Studies of the Institute for Family, Community, and Opportunity at The Heritage

Foundation and a medical student at Georgetown University. O'Shea is a practicing surgeon and a senior fellow in the Center for Health Policy Studies. Their report summarized the matter as follows:

a) "The unfunded mandatory adoption of the latest International Classification of Diseases (ICD-10) will add to the already considerable financial and administrative burdens on physician practices. Most physicians believe that ICD-10 will adversely impact healthcare and do not support its implementation. In fact, according to a 2014 Physicians Foundation Survey (September 2014), more than 75 percent of doctors believe it will needlessly complicate coding; more than 50 percent believe it will create 'severe' administrative problems; and 38 percent believe it will expose physicians to more liability—while only 11 percent think it will improve diagnosis and quality of care.

b) "The additional coding detail of ICD-10 will not help the physician treating that patient, since doctors do not treat according to diagnostic code, but according to the patient's clinical situation. Physicians will spend 15 percent more time working on documentation.

c) "Not only is implementation of ICD-10 codes a crushing burden on physicians, but also it is straining the much-needed vital resources to invest in new healthcare delivery models and well-developed technology that promotes care coordination with real value to the patient."

ICD-10 Coding—An Asset to Hospitals

However, the ICD-10 coding system is a boon to hospitals and owners of larger clinics because it allows them to link multiple, complex medical conditions to the original diagnosis. If a patient has neuropathy, for example, a physician may indicate connections to other conditions, such as diabetes, obesity, neurotoxic medications, and nutritional deficiencies. These notes in the patient's medical records make it possible to bill for as many clinical problems as possible, thus increasing the payments that owners receive from Medicare, Medicaid, or insurance companies.

Trisha was now required not only to record her patients' symptoms and the details of their physical examinations but also to enter their current medications, order appropriate tests, and complete the ICD-10 coding for billing. Even though almost all of the patients she was now seeing in the clinic were already Medicare-capitated patients, the submitted codes were used to justify a higher capitated level of payment from Medicare.

An example of such documentation of just the diagnosis, associated with the simultaneous presence of two chronic diseases or conditions in a patient, is listed below. This is from an actual follow-up patient, randomly selected by Trisha (it contains none of the patient's identifying information). It's easy to see how complicated and frustrating all of this record keeping becomes when the physician has only fifteen minutes to examine and care for a patient, as well as fill out line after line of detailed information.

> Diagnosis and Wrap-up:
> 1. Chronic kidney disease due to type 2 diabetes mellitus - A1c 7/20 - 6.7% - pt denies hypoglycemia. Continue insulin at 11 units bid subQ. Continue diet and exercise.
> 2. E11.22: Type 2 diabetes mellitus with diabetic chronic kidney disease
> 3. Dependence on hemodialysis due to end stage renal disease - Continue hemodialysis M, W, F. Continue to f/u with Dr. XXX
> 4. Z99.2: Dependence on renal dialysis
>   a. Rena-Vite 0.8 mg tablet -
> 5. Take 1 tablet(s) every day by oral route for 90 days. Qty: 90 tablet(s)   Refills: 3 Pharmacy: XXX

*6. Hypertensive heart AND chronic kidney disease on dialysis -
Continue Carvedilol. Continue Amlodipine*
7. N18.9: Chronic kidney disease, unspecified
*8. Long-term current use of insulin – Continue insulin. Diabetic
diet and exercise discussed.*
9. Z79.4: Long term (current) use of insulin
*10. Hyperlipidemia - Labs noted. 7/20 - Lipids controlled. Continue
Atorvastatin. Diet and exercise.*
11. E78.5: Hyperlipidemia, unspecified
        a. Atorvastatin 40 mg tablet -
*12. Take 1 tablet(s) every day by oral route for 90 days.   Qty: 90
tablet(s)   Refills: 1   Pharmacy: XXX*
        *a. HIGH CHOLESTEROL: CARE INSTRUCTIONS
GIVEN*
13. Mild recurrent major depression - Controlled on Sertraline
14. F33.0: Major depressive disorder, recurrent, mild
        a. Sertraline 50 mg tablet -
*15. Take 1 tablet(s) every day by oral route for 90 days. Qty: 90
tablet(s)   Refills: 1   Pharmacy: XXX*
        *a. DEPRESSION TREATMENT: CARE INSTRUCTIONS
GIVEN*
16. Finding of body mass index
*17. Z68.24: Body mass index (BMI) 24.0-24.9, adult dialysis due to
end stage renal disease - Continue hemodialysis M, W, F. Continue
to f/u with Dr. XXX*

Too Much to Do; Not Enough Time to Do It

All of Trisha's patients are cherry-picked by her clinic administrator because of their multiple medical issues. These are
sick patients who require more time and attention from their
doctors than the regularly scheduled time for each patient. To
enter the entire care data and billing codes in a patient's EHR
in the allocated fifteen minutes is not humanly possible. As a
result, the physician is late for the next patient, and this
vicious cycle continues. Between patients, Trisha reviews and
acts on fifty laboratory results from patients she has previous-
ly seen in the clinic, receives and answers fifteen telephone
messages from patients, writes out fifteen pharmacy prescriptions, and squeezes an additional one or two "emergency"
patients into her schedule.

All of the above work has to be recorded in each patient's EHR. Because the owner of the medical clinic wants to make sure that the maximum amount of money allowable is collected, Trisha receives at least ten messages a day from billing coders, via the patient's EHR, to edit, correct, and add relevant, additional diagnoses where possible. She is constantly reminded to focus on Medicare Risk Assessment factors and how "important" it is to record them in the chart. The more complex these factors are, the larger the reimbursement from Medicare.

The day's work doesn't end when Trisha returns home at seven in the evening. After dinner, she boots up her laptop and tries to finish as much of the day's work as possible. She usually puts in about three hours of work after dinner, almost every day. On weekends, she logs in eight hours a day in an attempt to catch-up on the previous week's work. Tricia is not paid for these extra hours.

Since the insurance company that owns the medical practice receives fixed income per patient per year, referral to a specialist for a second opinion or further care is considered a "financial drain" and is thus strongly discouraged. In, fact referring patients to specialists is closely monitored and grounds for a reprimand. Trisha remembers being summoned to the medical director's office because of her "excessive" referral pattern. She was put on three months' probation to correct the problem by making fewer referrals to specialists. She compiled a list of all the patients she had referred to various specialists and showed it to her medical director at her three-month, follow-up evaluation. Not a single patient on the list had been referred inappropriately.

Some had cancer and were referred to an oncologist, some had significant cardiac issues and were referred to a cardiologist, and so on. Trisha' medical director, while acknowledging that she had acted properly, gave her this advice: "I totally agree with you, but just between the two of us, I am asked by our employer to talk to you. To protect your employment and your career, you should drastically cut back on your referrals."

The Business Side of Healthcare

The medical director's employment and career also depend on how he or she, and other physicians, perform in the clinic under the medical director's management. Healthcare is a business to clinic owners; their ultimate goal is to make a profit. At the end of the year, when Trisha received her annual bonus, she was shocked to see that the check was for only $900. The clinic administrator justified the reduced bonus because of the "reduced value" Trisha was bringing to the organization, based in part to her referral pattern to specialists.

This travesty is not only happening to Trisha. Other physicians across the country report similar abuses. The problem is getting worse. I have heard over and over again from many physicians that "it is our own fault because we let this happen to us. We empowered administrators to push us around." They may be right. Physicians do their best at what they spent so many years learning to do—take care of patients.

Gradually and systematically, as hospitals, insurance companies, and healthcare administrators became more organized, their powerful lobby succeeded in having Congress design parts of the ACA to favor their interests. As a result, they have slowly but surely taken control of doctors, who are now their direct employees.

Administrators regulate how much money doctors can make per relative value unit (RVU)—a method for calculating the volume of work or effort expended by a physician in treating patients, the hours they must work, how many referrals they can make, and to whom. If they do make referrals to specialists, they are expected to use specialists who are "within the system." At the same time, insurance companies decide what tests and medications physicians can order,

These decisions, which are made without physician input, become mandatory policy. There is no mechanism for disagreement or appeal. Since physicians are legally prohibited from collective bargaining, this gives government regulators, hospitals, and insurance companies a distinct advantage and virtually ties the hands of doctors. They are asked to take on tasks that have nothing to do with caring for patients and could easily be handled by other personnel. It does not require a medical degree to enter ICD-10 codes and many other outcome measures; nonetheless, these are mandatory parts of physicians' job descriptions. While it doesn't seem reasonable that having physicians do clerical work would save money, in fact, it is. If clerical staff work even one extra hour a day, they would have to be paid time-and-a-half for overtime; whereas, no matter how many extra hours physicians put in, they are not paid for that time. Hour by hour, that adds up to a more robust bottom line for the clinic or hospital's bottom line.

The High Price of Fighting City Hall

Trisha was getting depressed. She had no time to see friends or family; she couldn't even squeeze in time to exercise. This situation surely was not the reason she had worked so hard and sacrificed so much to become a doctor. When I saw her, she was exhibiting all the signs of abuse. I asked her if she ever thought about taking legal actions against her employer. While her answer didn't surprise me, it made me sad.

"I thought about it," she said. "But fighting a giant company is draining, both financially and emotionally. Besides, I have a medical-school loan to pay, and I am bound by a twenty-mile radius non-compete clause in my contract. It is also difficult to be hired by another corporation if I come across as a 'trouble maker.' But, more importantly, I would lose all my patients with whom I have developed an emotional bond. My patients are what keep me going." Her only other alternative—private, solo practice—is not a viable option in today's healthcare environment.

Trisha's salary was fixed. She was not paid based on RVUs or how many patients she saw. So, it was to her employer's advantage to have her squeeze more patients into her schedule. The more patients she saw, the more money the practice earned. Since her clinic was always filled with Medicare patients, there were no slots left for her other patients. Officially, she was still their physician, but she had no time to see them. Because they were not seen on a regular basis, they called frequently for prescription refills and other medical issues, requests Tricia had to fill on her own time. Trisha felt uncomfortable prescribing medications without seeing the patients, sometimes for more than a year. Technically and legally, she was obligated to take care of them.

The relationship between a physician and patient can only be terminated with the consent of both parties; otherwise, the physician can be sued for "patient abandonment." Until proper notice is given, a physician is required to answer that patient's calls and attend to his or her medical needs.

The messages from her patients would come by way of "My Chart" in her EHR in-basket. If she didn't reply to them expediently, she would be reprimanded by administrators for having "incomplete medical records." This would, of course, be recorded in her personnel file and eventually affect her year-end bonus, something she had already experienced. "There is no other profession I know of that does so much work without being justly compensated," Trisha told me.

I agree with her because, recently, I got a $500 bill from my lawyer, whom I had called simply to inquire when I could expect an answer to an issue he was working on for me. Attorneys bill for every minute of their time; physicians, on the other hand, are expected to answer patient calls at odd hours, order tests, and prescribe medications without billing or being paid.

Recently, I was on call for our medical group. It was a busy night with patients calling all night with their medical issues and, as a result, I didn't get to bed until 2:00am. The following day was going to be a busy one at the clinic, so I went to work at 7:30 the next morning. I didn't get home until 8:00 that night. After dinner, I stayed up late to be with family, knowing that I should have uninterrupted sleep that night since I was not on call.

However, I was awakened at 4:00am from a sound sleep by a call from my answering service because an emergency-room physician, who had a question about a patient of mine, insisted on talking to me. The issue was not an urgent one, but it ruined my night. I couldn't get back to sleep again. This is not a rare instance. It happens all the time to other physicians around the country who cannot bill the patient for such services rendered. It was happening to Trisha several times a week, even when she was not on call.

The Lopsided Legal System

Trisha finally reached her breaking point. With no control over her schedule and an increasing amount of work, she found herself being "blackmailed" for referring patients to specialists when she deemed it medically necessary. Her priority was her patients' medical needs. In the event that a patient suffered because of a non-referral or even a delay in being referred to a specialist, Trisha was legally liable. Conversely, her employer, which happened to be a large healthcare insurance company, would be exempt from any meaningful liability. Current laws protect healthcare insurance companies from any wrongdoing but do not protect physicians.

According to Dr. Richard Roberts in an article in *Family Practice Management* (2003, 10(3): 29-34), non-referral to specialists in a timely manner is one of the seven top reasons family physicians are sued. More than the fear of being sued, Trisha's concern was that her patients would not receive the best possible care.

Clinics are huge money-making businesses. Care of patients takes a backseat to the amount of money they can earn. While employed physicians are paid less and less, clinic owners make more and more. Roughly one thousand companies provide managed healthcare to the majority of patients in the United States.

The CEOs of these health-insurance companies earn from several hundred thousand to millions of dollars per year, while an increasing number of people in this country struggle to afford basic healthcare. According to *Business Week*, an average CEO of a major health insurance company in 1980 made forty-two times an average hourly worker's pay. This doubled to eighty-five times average pay in 1990. In 2000, the average CEO's salary reached an unbelievable 531 times that of the average hourly worker!

Performance-based incentives and compensation linked to the overall financial success of the company are the driving forces behind a rigorous protocol that denies medical therapy in many situations, even when the treating doctor feels such therapy is medically necessary. The ever-increasing take-home pay for CEOs reflects that they are effective in controlling costs and increasing their revenue. This is a business. If they run it profitably, CEOs benefit; this is one of the reasons they are so highly paid.

CEOs feel protected because HMOs and health insurance companies are, for all practical purposes, immune to patients' lawsuits. This was the only industry exempt from such lawsuits until banks joined it in 2010, in the wake of the recession. In 1987, insurance industry lawyers were successful in convincing the US Supreme Court to have the federal Employee Retirement Income Security Act of 1974 (ERISA) put the healthcare industry above state common law, thus making it impossible to hold the industry accountable for its acts. If a patient who is denied doctor-recommended care by his HMO tries to file a case in a state court, where damages are available under that state's common law, HMO lawyers will have the case transferred to federal court under ERISA's rules. HMOs or insurers that lose the federal ERISA grievance only pay the cost of the procedure or benefits the patients were denied in the first place. There are no other damages or penalties.

What is fascinating is that companies are required to provide the benefit *only* when a patient survives long enough to receive it. If the patient dies before receiving the *prescribed* treatment, the insurer or HMO pays *nothing*. Because there is no meaningful penalty for denying medically necessary treatment, there is no good reason to approve any therapy that HMOs and insurance companies consider a financial drain.

Hijacking the Healthcare System

In 1991, there was a well-publicized case involving Mrs. Phyllis Cannon, who died because her insurance company refused to pay for an approved bone-marrow transplant therapy. The company invoked the ERISA ruling and, as a result, her husband received no compensation. The judges, however, were sympathetic and acknowledged the fact that the insurance company was clearly in the wrong for not approving the lifesaving therapy for Mrs. Cannon. But the law, they lamented, gave Mr. Cannon no remedy for his loss.

There is no remedy for Trisha's patients, either. Physicians who dare to advocate for their patients are effectively silenced by being fired or having their year-end bonuses reduced. Gone are the days when physicians had the time and the will to fight back. Treatment choices are governed by clerks or nurses who override the medical recommendations of treating physicians. The agony and frustration at this gross injustice is well captured in a statement made by a woman named Florence B. Corcoran, whose full-term baby died *in utero* because her insurance company denied her appropriate and much-needed medical care.

"If I go out on the street and murder a person, I am thrown in jail for murder and held accountable," said Ms. Corcoran. "What's the difference between me and this clerk, thousands of miles away, making a decision that took the life of my baby? The difference is that she gets off scot-free and keeps her job!"

This is only one example how the healthcare and insurance industries have hijacked the way healthcare is delivered and paid for in this country. Bad as it sounds, however, this would not be a hopeless situation if Congress took appropriate action. Congress has the power to change the healthcare scenario by focusing on two important issues: 1) directing and regulating the pharmaceutical industry to price drugs appropriately; and 2) holding insurance companies accountable for refusing to pay for therapies, tests, and procedures ordered by physicians. However, the powerful pharmaceutical and insurance lobbies have stood in the way of any progress on these two fronts.

As a result, here is an example of what often happens. I have been taking care of a young man who is a husband and father of two and whose generalized discomfort and weakness rendered him totally disabled. Extensive evaluation at the Mayo Clinic led to a bad-news-good-news-bad-news story. The bad news was a diagnosis of a rare autoimmune disorder. The good news was that his condition would improve with intravenous gamma globulin therapy, which it did. The bad news was that his condition regressed when his insurance company refused to cover his therapies.

My multiple letters and peer-to-peer conference calls with the insurance company's medical doctor were to no avail. Frustrated, I decided to get another opinion from a professor at the University of Chicago, who is internationally recognized for his expertise in this rare disorder. He recommended the same therapy I had prescribed.

Armed with letters from the professor and Mayo Clinic, I appealed to the insurance company to approve my patient's therapy. My request was once again refused, and my patient remains disabled and unable to work. We have hit a dead end and can see no other options. Knowing that he could improve if his therapy were approved by his insurance company and being denied that approval is, in my opinion, a crime.

If this were an isolated case, that would be bad enough. But, sadly, there are thousands of such patients who are refused the care that would turn their lives around. This is a situation Congress could change if it chooses to take action.

Not too long ago, one of my patients was admitted to the hospital because of a stroke. I reviewed her chart and asked her why she was not taking the stroke-prevention drug, Plavix, I had prescribed for her after her previous mini-stroke. She was silent for a moment and then tearfully explained: "Doctor, either my husband gets his heart medicine, or I get my Plavix because we can't afford both." On fixed Social Security income, they couldn't pay for the exorbitantly expensive drugs. The irony is that these same drugs, manu-factured by the same pharmaceutical companies, cost a fraction of the price in other countries. Congress could not only rein in drug prices but also make sure that insurance companies pay for the necessary drugs. Why do insurance companies cover all but a tiny fraction of a $100,000 hospitali-zation but ask patients to pay 20 percent or more of the cost of a life-saving $100,000 cancer drug?

As a physician who specializes in caring for patients with MS, I marvel at the therapeutic advances made for this illness in the last two decades. We now have fourteen different FDA-approved therapies for patients with MS. However, the health -insurance companies restrict our progress by approving payment for only a select number of these therapies.

The selection of therapies is guided by "rebates received" from the pharmaceutical companies, according to a number of drug-industry officials I interviewed recently. It is well known that one year, an insurance company may designate a particular drug as "preferred" (Tier 1 on its formulary), only to drop it the following year in favor of another, similar drug that had been declared "non-preferred" the previous year. There is no justifiable reason for the switch, since there have been no new studies to show any difference in efficacy or side effects.

Patients Lose, Big Pharma Wins

Politicians make noise when the actions of the pharmaceutical industry cause public outrage, but they do nothing concrete about it. While lawmakers are quick to pass laws that govern healthcare providers because of a lack of any collective resistance, "Big Pharma" continues to pour millions of dollars into lobbying Congress.

The EpiPen saga exemplifies what has become a routine in this country. Americans were outraged by a 500-percent increase in the price of a lifesaving EpiPen injection—from $100 in 2009 to $608 for a pack of two injections in 2016. The active medicine, however, should not cost more than $1 per injection. As parents struggled to obtain this life-saving medicine for their children, the CEO of that pharmaceutical company enjoyed a 671-percent increase in her salary. She correctly stated that her salary of $18.9 million in total compensation in 2015 was not excessive for the industry.

Daraprim, a lifesaving drug for certain patients with AIDS, was developed some sixty years ago, yet the pharmaceutical company that recently bought the rights to Daraprim, promptly (and legally) increased the price from $13.50 per tablet to $750 per tablet—a five thousand percent escalation! What is disturbing is the blatant statement by Turing Pharmaceuticals CEO Martin Shkreli that "the drug is not overpriced compared to its peers"—drawing attention to the fact that price hiking is the industry norm. While physicians wrote to the company urging them to reconsider the pricing since it would be impossible for the majority of AIDS patients who need this drug to come up with half-a-million dollars, the politicians who have the power to do something and save lives simply gave lip service to the issue until it faded from the headlines.

Huge salaries for pharmaceutical, insurance, and healthcare administrators have become the industry standard. They keep increasing each year, whereas physicians are making less or having to work more to maintain their income. This is difficult for physicians to handle, especially after spending so many years in school and sacrificing so much to become doctors.

This is only one of many sources of stress. Another is being told how to practice medicine, not for the sake of patients but rather to produce profits for the owners of their practices. Yet another major stressor is ICD-10, a statistical process that does nothing to improve the quality of care of patients yet takes a disproportionate amount of time to complete for each patient doctors see. Not only is it required for billing insurance companies, but it must also be associated with each of the tests ordered per patient in order to be adequately reimbursed by insurance carriers.

ICD-10 Coding—Time Consuming, Complicated, Counterproductive

Trisha explained it further: "In order for insurance companies to authorize an MRI of a brain in a patient in whom you are only 'suspecting' MS, you have to put down the diagnosis as MS because there is no ICD-10 code for 'possible' MS. Simply putting in symptoms would never get the MRI approved by the insurance company. Once you enter a 'diagnosis' to get the MRI approved, it is impossible to remove it from the patient's EHR, even though that 'diagnosis' is no longer correct. In the extra time it takes to attend to ICD-10 codes for all my patients in a day," she adds, "I could easily see a couple of extra patients or spend more time with the patients I do see." EHRs have built-in ICD-10 codes, which force me to comply. Otherwise, the program does not let me finish the patient's 'chart' or successfully order the tests I need for my other patients."

Migraine affects about 12 percent of Americans and is a common condition seen in clinic by neurologists. Recently, I ordered an MRI scan of the brain on EPIC (an EHR software for mid-size and large medical groups, hospitals, and integrated healthcare organizations) for one of my migraine patients. It was very easy until EPIC asked me to enter the patient's diagnosis. It would not accept simply migraine. I was required to go through more than seventy-five codes (see below) and select the appropriate code before EPIC would accept my MRI order. Not only was it time consuming, it was also very frustrating because it did nothing to change how I would manage my patient's care.

Software required that the author go through more than 75 ICD-10 codes and select the appropriate code before EPIC would accept his MRI order.

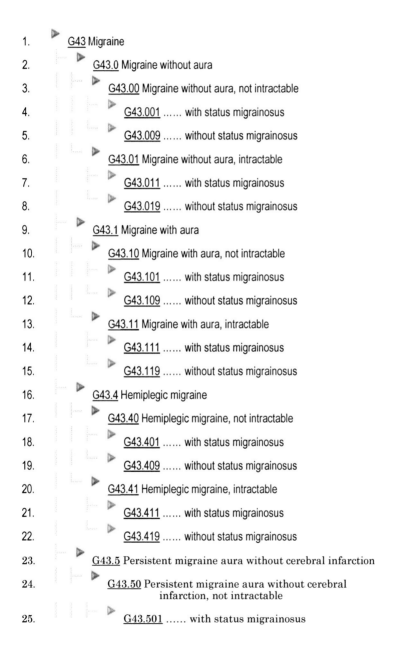

1. G43 Migraine
2. G43.0 Migraine without aura
3. G43.00 Migraine without aura, not intractable
4. G43.001 …… with status migrainosus
5. G43.009 …… without status migrainosus
6. G43.01 Migraine without aura, intractable
7. G43.011 …… with status migrainosus
8. G43.019 …… without status migrainosus
9. G43.1 Migraine with aura
10. G43.10 Migraine with aura, not intractable
11. G43.101 …… with status migrainosus
12. G43.109 …… without status migrainosus
13. G43.11 Migraine with aura, intractable
14. G43.111 …… with status migrainosus
15. G43.119 …… without status migrainosus
16. G43.4 Hemiplegic migraine
17. G43.40 Hemiplegic migraine, not intractable
18. G43.401 …… with status migrainosus
19. G43.409 …… without status migrainosus
20. G43.41 Hemiplegic migraine, intractable
21. G43.411 …… with status migrainosus
22. G43.419 …… without status migrainosus
23. G43.5 Persistent migraine aura without cerebral infarction
24. G43.50 Persistent migraine aura without cerebral infarction, not intractable
25. G43.501 …… with status migrainosus

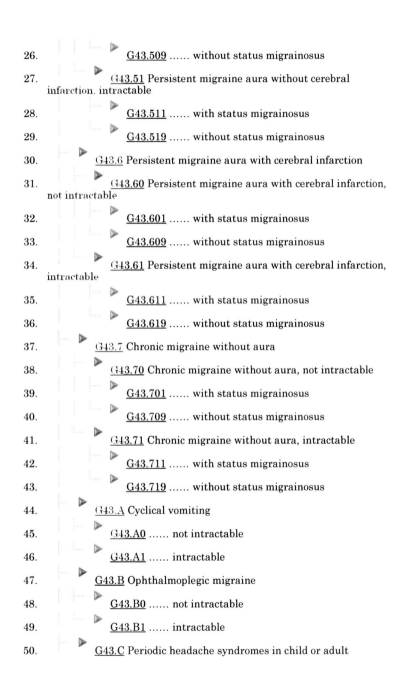

26. G43.509 ...... without status migrainosus

27. G43.51 Persistent migraine aura without cerebral infarction, intractable

28. G43.511 ...... with status migrainosus

29. G43.519 ...... without status migrainosus

30. G43.6 Persistent migraine aura with cerebral infarction

31. G43.60 Persistent migraine aura with cerebral infarction, not intractable

32. G43.601 ...... with status migrainosus

33. G43.609 ...... without status migrainosus

34. G43.61 Persistent migraine aura with cerebral infarction, intractable

35. G43.611 ...... with status migrainosus

36. G43.619 ...... without status migrainosus

37. G43.7 Chronic migraine without aura

38. G43.70 Chronic migraine without aura, not intractable

39. G43.701 ...... with status migrainosus

40. G43.709 ...... without status migrainosus

41. G43.71 Chronic migraine without aura, intractable

42. G43.711 ...... with status migrainosus

43. G43.719 ...... without status migrainosus

44. G43.A Cyclical vomiting

45. G43.A0 ...... not intractable

46. G43.A1 ...... intractable

47. G43.B Ophthalmoplegic migraine

48. G43.B0 ...... not intractable

49. G43.B1 ...... intractable

50. G43.C Periodic headache syndromes in child or adult

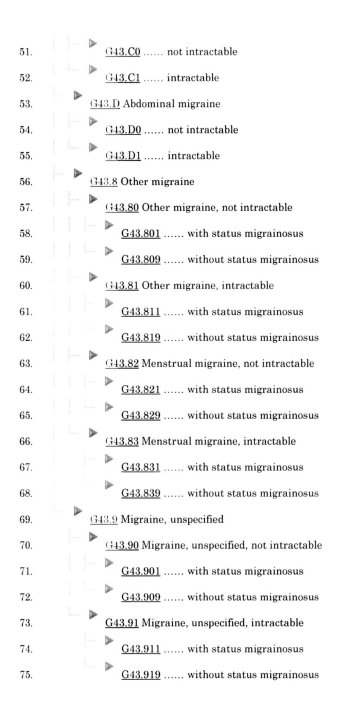

51. G43.C0 ...... not intractable

52. G43.C1 ...... intractable

53. G43.D Abdominal migraine

54. G43.D0 ...... not intractable

55. G43.D1 ...... intractable

56. G43.8 Other migraine

57. G43.80 Other migraine, not intractable

58. G43.801 ...... with status migrainosus

59. G43.809 ...... without status migrainosus

60. G43.81 Other migraine, intractable

61. G43.811 ...... with status migrainosus

62. G43.819 ...... without status migrainosus

63. G43.82 Menstrual migraine, not intractable

64. G43.821 ...... with status migrainosus

65. G43.829 ...... without status migrainosus

66. G43.83 Menstrual migraine, intractable

67. G43.831 ...... with status migrainosus

68. G43.839 ...... without status migrainosus

69. G43.9 Migraine, unspecified

70. G43.90 Migraine, unspecified, not intractable

71. G43.901 ...... with status migrainosus

72. G43.909 ...... without status migrainosus

73. G43.91 Migraine, unspecified, intractable

74. G43.911 ...... with status migrainosus

75. G43.919 ...... without status migrainosus

Entering all of this information has done nothing to improve the quality of care for our patients. In fact, it has had the opposite effect by reducing the time we have to spend with them. By itself, coding may not seem such a big deal, but it is only one of many administrative duties that take physicians away from our primary responsibility—bonding with and listening to our patients. That shortchanges patients and takes a toll on physicians. In the end, ICD-10 coding is a zero-sum game: whatever administrators gain financially by instituting the practice is offset by what both patients and doctors lose.

I am not suggesting that recording diagnoses, medications, therapies, and other pertinent patient information is a useless endeavor. There may be great value in the future in terms of spotting trends and conducting research, but it has no direct benefit for patients at the moment. As I have said, administrative work takes an inordinate amount of time, puts unnecessary pressure on physicians, and infringes on the doctor-patient relationship.

EHR has cut down by 50 percent the number of patients we can see in a day, and it hardly makes use of the skills we have to offer. It would be far more practical and cost effective to hire a data-entry person to do what they are trained to do and let physicians do what we are trained to do. Why that hasn't occurred to the hospital and insurance companies that own medical practices remains a mystery.

EHR has a number of drawbacks, many of which physicians have learned to live with, but none is as onerous as ICD-10 Codes. Perhaps I would change my opinion *if* they improved the quality of care we give our patients, which they do not; *if* they allowed us to see more patients in a day, which they do not; *if* they made it easier to arrive at a simple diagnosis, which they do not; or *if* they enabled us to observe and bond with our patients, which they do not. In addition to all of this "coding," physicians are asked to do many other unrelated tasks, all of which rob us of our autonomy and patients of our undivided attention in the examining room.

Chapter 5

Physician Burnout:
The Problem Nobody Talks About

*"The physical and emotional health of an entire generation and the
economic health and security of our nation are at stake."*
—Former First Lady Michelle Obama

K arl was ready. He had been training for over twelve
years and now, at age thirty-four, he felt he could
win the competition. As a personal trainer for fifteen
years, he had motivated and helped hundreds of people not
only to get physically fit but also to live healthier lifestyles.
He believed the key to success was to encourage his clients to
think and act outside their comfort zones.

"Great things can be achieved that way. By nature, your
body wants to conserve energy and is very happy to stay in
that comfort zone, but your mind knows better!" Karl told me
as we sat down to talk over a hot bowl of protein-rich, vegan
chili soup one afternoon. "Once your mind is motivated, your
body has to listen, and you can then sculpt your body the way
you want it to look."

Karl had done just that. He had chiseled every muscle in
his body to achieve perfection. Years of discipline, daily
workouts, and a well-balanced diet had achieved his desired
outcome. He was in ideal shape and ready for the bodybuilding competition that was to take place the following day.

As he was crossing the road to get to a shopping mall, he visualized himself on the stage, receiving his championship trophy. He could literally hear the crowd going wild and clapping. But, at that moment, he was suddenly flung high in the air by a speeding car and hit the concrete pavement with a loud thud. The first thing Karl remembers was being loaded into an ambulance.

"Do not give me any salt! I am competing in a bodybuilding exhibition tomorrow," he told the paramedics as they put the tourniquet on his arm and prepped him to insert an intravenous line. One of the paramedics, who was in touch with the ER over the radio, told them that the patient was moving all of his extremities but was delirious. Karl now really panicked, insisting that he was not delirious. He blurted out the date, the name of the current US president, and where his competition was going to take place.

Karl knew that water and sodium were the trickiest elements to manage during the pre-contest period. Water can accumulate in the subcutaneous fluid and obscure muscle striations, much like a thin layer of body fat. Blood sodium concentration is equally important. Because competitive bodybuilders are aware that high-serum sodium levels lead to greater water retention, they start restricting sodium consumption weeks before and severely curtailing it the day before the contest. He didn't want the IV salt solution the paramedics were about to give him. They were puzzled, but honored his request once he signed a piece of paper indicating that he was going against their medical advice.

By the time he arrived at the ER, both his legs were numb, but he could still move them well. Multiple CT scans of his head and spine failed to reveal any abnormities. The doctors cleaned and sutured his multiple wounds and sent him home, instructing him to follow-up with a spine specialist. Reassured that there were no spinal fractures or blood clots in his brain, Karl focused on the following day's contest. He had worked hard for this day and had been mentally and physically as fit as possible—until this accident.

Now, his entire body ached, both his legs were numb, and sharp pains radiated from his lower back down into his legs. Flat on his back, he wondered whether he would be able to compete the following day. Posing and holding his muscles in a contracted position to show his best physical form was a painful and strenuous process. What if his muscles cramped up, which would be even more painful. If that happened, he would be forced to drop out.

After a few minutes, his eyes welling up with tears, Karl's gaze landed on a framed poster of Lance Armstrong, which he had hung on the wall opposite his bed some years ago. He had read its message a hundred times, but now he felt that each of the words on the poster was addressing him directly. "Pain is temporary. If I quit now, it will last forever." The words had a profound effect on him. Some powerful force stirred his consciousness. He sharpened his focus and, at that moment, resolved to participate in the competition.

"Mind over matter," he kept telling himself. To achieve greatness, he had to move beyond his mental and physical blocks.

Early the following morning, Karl showed up for the competition for pre-judging. Despite his sutured wounds and pain, he participated in the contest, and he won big time—in every category. He was the overall champion! Elated, he felt he could now make his clients truly believe what he had only been preaching thus far! "You can achieve anything, if you really want it, and if you are willing to step outside your comfort zone."

However, Karl's low-back pain continued to worsen and, eventually, he saw a neurologist. An MRI revealed a large protruding disc that was compressing the nerves as they exited the lumbar spine. A consultation with an orthopedic surgeon was set up. After examining Karl and looking at his MRI scans, the surgeon recommended that he should quit lifting anything more than fifteen pounds and stop exercising. The doctor arranged for Karl to have an epidural steroid injection and prescribed strong narcotics to control his pain.

As Karl sat before this surgeon, who easily weighed over 350 pounds and struggled to get up from his chair, he couldn't help but ask himself the question, "Why should I listen to this doctor who cannot even take care of himself?" Karl asked if he could do some exercises that would not put a strain on his back. The answer was very straightforward: "Do not lift any weights for six months." If the pain didn't subside by then, surgery would be required.

Karl left his office, got in his car, and drove straight to the gym. He started to exercise, first with "baby weights" and then gradually increasing the intensity and the weights. He did just the opposite of what the orthopedic surgeon had advised him to do. Five months later, he deadlifted 605 pounds and won first place in a statewide dead-lifting championship.

Karl continues to inspire his clients to achieve better health and to exercise regularly. When I asked him if he sees a doctor on a regular basis, he said something very important, which I strongly believe every physician should hear: "Physicians should instill trust, respect, and comfort in you by the way they look and carry themselves. They should practice what they preach. Most of them are not walking the walk."

The Consequences of Obesity

Enough research exists to support Karl's statement. Healthcare providers who do not look healthy and appear out of shape fail to inspire healthy lifestyles in their patients. On the other hand, doctors who look fit and in shape do have a positive influence on their patients. In a study published in the *International Journal of Obesity* (2013), Dr. Rebecca Puhl and her colleagues reported that providers' excess weight may negatively affect patients' perceptions of their credibility, level of trust, and inclination to follow medical advice.

As Karl said, you should be in a position to confidently look into your clients' eyes to convince them of whatever you are asking them to do. According to a recent Johns Hopkins study by Gatz and Gaglani, "Despite their knowledge of the dangers of chronic disease killers from unhealthy lifestyles, roughly six in ten doctors and nurses today are overweight or obese, a level approaching that in the general population."

Obesity is defined as excess adipose tissue (loose connective tissue in which fat cells accumulate), which produces a number of different pro-inflammatory toxins, leading to various medical problems, including cardio-vascular disease and diabetes. The diagnosis of obesity is based on body mass index (BMI), derived from a formula that compares weight to height.

BMI converts a person's tissue mass (muscle, fat, bones) into a value and categorizes that value as underweight, normal weight, overweight, or obese. A healthy BMI ranges from 19 to 25. Calculating BMI requires using the metric system to turn weight from pounds into kilograms and inches into centimeters. Here are the steps:

a) Step 1: Multiply your weight in pounds by 0.45 (the metric conversion factor to kilograms).

b) Step 2: Multiply your height in inches by 0.025 (the metric conversion factor to centimeters).

c) Step 3: Square your height (in centimeters).

d) Step 4: Divide your weight (in kg) by your height (in cm) squared.

Let's use Mary as an example. Mary is 5'7" and 132 pounds. Step 1 converts pounds into kilograms (132 lbs. x 0.45 = 59.4 kg). Step 2 converts her height in inches to centimeters (67 in x 0.025 = 1.675 cm). Step 3 squares the height (1.675 x 1.675 = 2.805). Step 4 divides weight by height squared (59.4 kg / 2.805 cm = 21.21). Mary's BMI is 21.2.

To determine what your BMI means, here is the scale: Underweight = <18.5; Normal weight = 18.5–24.9; overweight = 25–29.9; obese = BMI of 30 or greater. In other words, if your BMI is 25 to 29.9, you are overweight but not obese. A BMI of thirty or more is in the obese range. The United States has the highest obesity rate in the world!

Obesity is the leading cause of mortality and disability in this country. It costs in excess of $190 billion a year to take care of the medical problems associated with obesity. Roughly 44 percent of diabetes, 23 percent of ischemic heart disease, and 7 to 41 percent of certain cancers are attributable to overweight and obesity. According to the Centers for Disease Control and Prevention (CDC), an estimated 112,000 deaths per year are associated with obesity, nationally.

The Physician-Burnout Crisis

The question is why aren't doctors taking care of themselves? Among the innumerable answers, the most important is the increasing rate of physician burnout. A national survey published in the *Archives of Family Medicine* in 2012 reported that close to half of all US physicians suffer from burnout—far more than other American workers. A recent study by the Mayo Clinic revealed that this crisis had reached a dangerous level. Stress is the leading culprit. Dealing with hospital administrators, insurance companies, declining payments for services rendered, pharma regulations, increasing malpractice lawsuits, and escalating overhead have contributed to the burnout crisis.

The level of unhappiness among physicians is on the rise, leading to a higher suicide rates than any other profession in this country. Chronic stress can wreak havoc on the mind and body. People who do not eat healthy food, exercise, or sleep well are at increased risk for numerous health problems.

Most physicians work more than ten hours a day, five days a week. They get home from work at around 7:00pm, spend some time with family during the evening meal, and then do unfinished work before going to sleep. There is no time for exercise or other recreational activities. If they have some free time, they spend it catching up with medical journals, which pile up over time. This unhealthy cycle continues and takes a toll on their physical well-being.

It is not surprising that depression and substance abuse are major problems among physicians. Every year, between three and four hundred doctors take their own lives—roughly one a day. No other profession has a higher suicide rate. Divorce rates are 10 to 20 percent higher than in the general population. Physicians are notorious for not seeking professional help when they need it. This is partly because they fear decreased respect by their peers and loss of referrals and income. A diagnosis of mental illness has to be self-reported, as well as reported by peers who are asked to submit a report every time the physician's staff privileges come up for renewal. This information is discussed at credential-committee meetings, the members of which are not to sworn to secrecy, so the word gets around easily.

What Doctors Can Do to Curb the Crisis

Despite the many stressors physicians must deal with, there is something they can do about the toll stress takes on their minds and bodies. To begin with, they can control their weight and avoid becoming obese. A reduced waist size leads to a longer life. Under the guidelines of the International Diabetes Federation, a normal waist line for a woman is thirty-two inches or less, and for a man it is thirty-eight inches or less. Men with a waist size greater than forty inches and women with a waist size greater than thirty-five inches are at increased risk for heart disease and stroke.

In a large study involving 33,193 men, Radim Jurca, an exercise physiologist at the Cooper Institute in Dallas, revealed that every two-inch increase in waist size raises the risk of dying within the next ten years of cardiovascular disease by up to 17 percent, independent of other risk factors. Many studies stress the importance of waistline and general health; in fact, every five inches that waist size exceeds the ideal target, the risk of dying from any cause increases by 20 to 40 percent.

A Mayo Clinic study that followed 13,000 subjects for fourteen years found that the risk of cardiovascular death was 2.75 times higher, and the risk of death from all causes was 2.08 times higher in people with above-average waistlines. (To measure your waist, stand in front of a mirror with your feet apart and wrap the tape around your waist just about an inch above your belly button. Breathe normally; don't hold your breath in.)

The good news is that physicians have the power to change their lifestyles and take charge of their health. As little as one hour a day, focused on making a few changes in behavior, can produce drastic changes in a person's health and vitality, which will enable doctors to better handle stress and more effectively fight burnout.

If He Can Do It, You Can Too!

Dr. Asish Trivedi, who ran a solo neurology practice in Seattle for fifteen years, put this theory to the test in his own life. Dr. Trivedi was heading toward burnout. The chronic stress related to an escalation in administrative duties was driving him crazy. He felt emotionally and physically drained and that he had nothing more to give as a physician. He was no longer excited about going to work in the morning. Every day was just another day. He was exhausted, and his threshold for losing his cool was beginning to concern him.

"It was perhaps okay and arguably acceptable to get angry at insurance companies and hospital administrators, but I knew it was a serious problem when it started to spill over to my patients, whom I dearly loved and respected!"

Dr. Trivedi had to do *something!* He refused to be one more number added to the physician-burnout crisis.

According to the most recent and important study conducted by Dr. Christine Sinsky and her colleagues (*Annals of Internal Medicine*, September 2016), physicians who worked in outpatient-care settings spent nearly two hours on clerical work for every one hour they dedicated to seeing patients during in clinic. Furthermore, only 27 percent of the total time spent with the patient was direct face-to-face time. The rest of the time was spent on the computer and desk duties—everything the physician has to do *after* the face-to-face time with the patient. The mandatory addition of EHR has made it necessary to spend a disproportionate amount of time interacting with the computer screen instead of the patient. For many physicians, this has caused extreme dissatisfaction and taken the joy out of practicing medicine.

All of this was weighing heavily on Dr. Trivedi's mind when he went to pick up his wife at a CrossFit gym. As he waited for the class to end, he caught a glimpse of a woman who was carrying heavy weights as she ran up a flight of the stairs. He was struck by her strength and vitality, and as she turned around to run in his direction, he was stunned. "Oh, my God! That's my wife," he blurted out. His wife had been trying for more than a year to get him to join the gym, but he had always brushed her off, saying he was quite active at his work and didn't need any more physical stress. But now, he was shocked by what his wife was able to do. He was impressed by how young and vibrant she looked on the gym floor, and right then, he made a decision.

From Sedentary to Strenuous

He joined the very next class that was to start in two hours. The first thing the trainer asked him to do was pull-ups. As he hung himself with his hands firmly around the bar and trying to thrust his body upwards, he realized that no matter how much he struggled, he couldn't move at all. With the trainer's help, pushing his legs upwards, he completed his first-ever pull-up.

The rest of the workout that day was a torture, but he struggled through every step of it. He remembers it all too well. "I was able to do less than one percent of what I was asked to do, but I felt really good after I was done. For the first time in a long time, I was sweating profusely; my sweat-soaked clothes never felt so good! I was elated, even though I had failed miserably. Before leaving the gym, all of my classmates patted me on my back and told me that they looked forward to seeing me again the following day."

After class, as he sat down for dinner, he actually felt *hungry*. He ate well and, to his wife's surprise, skipped his daily *must-have* dessert. That night, he recalls, he slept better than he had in a long time. Even his clinic staff commented how well he looked the following morning. He knew he was on the right path. Dr. Trivedi had found the way to escape burnout. He couldn't wait to get to the gym, and now, five years later, he still can't wait. He is there every day, six days a week. Everyone now knows that from 6:00 to 7:30pm, the doctor is working out at the gym.

He is an inspiration to others in the class as he does a hundred pull-ups in just a few minutes. In the beginning, he struggled to do a hand-stand even with support, but now he does thirty hand-stand pushups without a problem. Within six months, he lost six inches off his waistline. He is now per-ceived in a whole new way by his family, friends, coworkers, and patients. One day, as he walked out of the bathroom shirtless, his daughter looked at him and said, "Dad, you have a six-pack!"

"Not too many fifty-year-old dads have a six-pack, said Dr. Trivedi, with a sense of pride. "Exercising has given me my life back! It saved me! As soon as I began to exercise and be around *health-conscious* people at the gym, I started to pay attention to my diet and eat better. For the first time, I calculated my protein, carbohydrate, and fat intake. It came naturally to me. One healthy change led to so many other healthy changes. Improvements in my diet seemed to go hand in hand with my exercise program.

"Being a strict vegetarian, it was a challenge to take in enough protein, but then I paid more attention to foods rich in protein. We ate healthier meals at home. Alcohol adversely affected my workouts, so now I rarely consume alcohol. A metamorphosis towards a better lifestyle was beginning to occur in our family, as well. I was much happier and more productive at work. The daily stress was there and, in fact, even worse with the Affordable Care Act, but I found myself handling it in a more positive way than I had in the past. My threshold for getting angry is much higher now. In the past, I would look at the clock and dread when I had ten more patients to see before the clinic ended at 5:00pm. But now, I liken it to a challenge I set up for myself to accomplish at the gym.

"The sense of achievement from doing a few more pushups, carrying heavier weights, and giving and receiving encouragement from my classmates gave me a lot of pride and contentment, which I was lacking at work all these years," explained Dr. Trivedi. "No matter how much I worked, the frustration of dealing with administrative work left me with a sense of emptiness. I did not choose to become a doctor to spend two hours of sitting in front of a computer doing clerical for every one hour I spent face to face with my patients. But, somehow, what I gained at the gym spilled over big time at work. It translated into much better relationship with my staff, my colleagues, and my patients. Now, I do not hesitate at all to add a few extra patients to my clinic. For me, it is no different than striving to do a few more pull-ups. It gives me a sense of fulfillment at the end of the day. Time goes by faster when I am happy, and I do a lot more work than I did before."

His colleagues at work noticed the difference in him as well and asked what he was doing differently. Surprised, they wanted to know when he found time to work out. "Finding time was a challenge for me at first," Dr. Trivedi admitted, "but I resolved to leave my office every day at 5:30pm and head straight to the gym. My clinic staff adjusted to my new routine and made sure I was able to get out in time. My patients also called earlier in the day with their concerns, rather than waiting until the last minute. In fact, most of my patients expressed their happiness for me, and some were even inspired to start exercising, themselves. 'If the doctor can find time, so can I,' they commented."

And that is exactly what Dr. Trivedi would say to his colleagues. "Despite being a solo practitioner, if *I* can find time to exercise, so can you! You owe this to yourself, to your family, and to your patients."

A Secondary Benefit of Exercise

One of the major benefits of working out at a gym is the wonderful team of friends and supporters he has developed over the years. For Dr. Trivedi, this is invaluable. He finds it refreshing to talk about non-medical topics with them. During the ninety minutes he spends in class, the doctor lets down his guard and talks like any other guy on the street. At the clinic, he has to be careful not use any *un*civilized language," but at the gym, he lets out his stress and utters a "few words" without any reservations.

A year after he joined the gym, one of the members asked him (pointing to his beeper), "Are you drug dealer or a plumber? No one else carries a beeper these days." When Dr. Trivedi disclosed his profession, the man was shocked and, in fact, refused to believe him because he said he had never before heard a doctor utter so many profanities!

When I recently talked to my friend, Karl, the body builder and fitness coach, about Dr. Trivedi, he smiled broadly and said, "Now that is one dude I would not mind having as my doctor!"

Exercise is the best way to fight burnout. In his inaugural address as the 162nd president of the American Medical Association in 2007, Dr. Ronald M. Davis, a physician who specialized in preventive medicine, emphasized this by stating that "exercise is medicine."

In fact, exercise is the most powerful tool we have to enhance the mind-body connection and to counter and heal the havoc of chronic stress. Human growth hormone (HGH), also known as a stress hormone, stimulates growth, cell reproduction, and cell regeneration and plays a crucial role in keeping our bodies trim and fit. HGH declines as we age and, by middle age, it is only 10 percent of what it is in early childhood. A sedentary lifestyle and chronic stress drastically inhibit the production of this hormone. On the other hand, recent research indicates that high-intensity exercises stimulate the production of HGH.

Dr. Trivedi found his fountain of youth with his intense exercise program. Not only did it help him physically, it also did wonders for his emotional well-being. Exercise triggered many physiological and psychological changes, which took him away from the self-destructive path he was heading down. Essentially, he healed himself. He now has a youthful spring in his walk, and his memory and concentration have improved as well. He noticed this recently while he was preparing for his specialty-board examinations. "One day, I must have spent more than twelve hours studying. I didn't move much at all from my desk, and I felt great! I could not have done that before. Even my daughter remarked that she had never seen me sit for so long without taking breaks every thirty to sixty minutes. And I scored higher than I ever had before in my board examinations."

Growing Your Brain

What Dr. Trivedi experienced is a direct effect of exercise on the brain. The human brain is made up of more than ten billion cells that control every function of the body, including memory. Each of the single cells is 0.0001 inch in diameter and has enough information in its DNA to fill one thousand books of six hundred pages each. The brain weighs about three pounds and, in a life span of seventy-five years, the brain works 24/7 for 657,000 hours. No computer exists that can come close to what the human brain can do. The brain is capable of producing conscious thoughts that can heal or destroy our bodies. According to William James, "(the) power to move the world is in your subconscious mind." The subconscious mind can do wonders for you if you know how to put it to use for overall benefits to your health.

Professor Eric Kandel at Columbia University, who was awarded 2000 Nobel Prize for his groundbreaking research in neuroscience, showed that exercise can help the brain grow new neurons and develop new synapses and connections, thus enhancing brain functions. More recently, using a 3T MRI scanner, a team of researchers headed by Dr. Teresa Liu-Ambrose, an associate professor in the Brain Research Center at the University of British Columbia, studied the effects of intense aerobic exercise on the size of the hippocampus. She reported in the *British Journal of Sports Medicine* (April 2014) that aerobic training significantly increased the size of the hippocampus, a part of brain that is involved in the formation of new memories, learning, and emotions.

This is an important finding because it is estimated that nearly 47 million people worldwide live with dementia. This number is expected to double in twenty years. With no reversible or preventive therapies available at present, the positive effects of exercise on memory are essential.

What is a beneficial amount of exercise? The American Heart Association recommends 150 minutes of moderate exercise or seventy-five minutes of vigorous exercise weekly. As a rule of thumb, thirty minutes a day, five times a week, of exercise leads to better overall cardiovascular health.

According to Professor Liu-Ambrose, "For the most robust brain health, it's probably advisable to incorporate both aerobic and resistance training. It seems that each type of exercise selectively targets different aspects of cognition, probably by sparking the release of different proteins in the body and brain."

This chapter has been a reminder of many things physicians have probably heard before, but sometimes it helps to hear familiar information more than once. Actions you can take to care for yourself, avoid burnout, and maintain a healthy lifestyle, see Chapter 10, "Physician, Heal Thyself."

Chapter 6

The Sunshine Act:
Shedding Light or Casting Shadows?

*"The principal villain in rising healthcare costs is the government. Not
pharmaceutical companies, not doctors, but government."*
—Neal Boortz. Author, attorney, and former Libertarian radio host

Angela had dreamed of this moment for many years.
The first cry of her newborn daughter made her
forget all the pain she had endured over the last
twenty-four hours. With the encouragement of her husband,
she clenched her teeth hard and, with all the strength she
could muster, gave one final push, bringing her daughter into
this world. She and her husband were elated and ready to
assume their role as parents.

Two days later, Angela experienced severe pain over her
left eye and lost vision in that eye. The OB/GYN was able to
get a neurologist to see her right away. The neurologist, who
examined Angela thoroughly, ordered an MRI of her brain
and cervical cord. The MRI revealed that both were highly
abnormal. Pointing to the big white spots on the MRI, the
doctor explained to Angela and her husband that she was
suffering from MS. He said that the presence of the contrast
dye in her cervical cord and left optic nerve meant that her
disease was active. He recommended intravenous steroids to
help her regain her vision.

Angela's vision did return to normal, and she had no other symptoms for a year, when she suddenly lost vision in her other eye. At the same time, her legs became so weak that she could hardly walk. She and her husband saw the same neurologist who had diagnosed her condition. He suspected that she was having a MS relapse. He ordered another MRI, which showed a worsening in the number and size of lesions in both the brain and spinal cord.

Angela was again put on steroids, which helped her vision, but did not affect the weakness in her legs. She began to use a walker to get around. It was difficult because her daughter had started to walk, and keeping up with her wasn't easy. She was happy that, at least, her vision had improved but not at all happy about gaining weight—a side effect of steroids. Eleven months later—two years after her initial diagnosis—Angela was bothered by memory problems and decided to come to our MS center for help.

This time, the MRI of the brain showed that her disease was getting worse. Walking with a walker across a room was a chore. I reviewed her medications and was very surprised to note that she had not received any preventative treatments. Numerous studies show the benefit of early treatment. Preventing relapses, which these drugs do very effectively, leads to less disability progression over time. "Relapses do matter," according to Dr. Fred Lublin in an interview by Grace Frank (*Multiple Sclerosis News Today*, 2016). "Relapses have long-term consequences. They cause cumulative disability, and this is very important for patients." Dr. Lublin, the Saunders Family Professor of Neurology and Director of the Corinne Goldsmith Dickenson Center for Multiple Sclerosis at Mount Sinai Medical Center in New York City, has been a prominent MS researcher whose work has shaped MS care around the world. There has been a growing concern among MS physicians that a delay in treatment usually results in patients becoming more disabled.

The Benefits of Early Treatment

The concept of "time is brain" (the sooner you treat the condition, the better the outcome) has prompted doctors not only to start a treatment early but also to escalate the therapy in the event that the current therapy does not give the desired outcomes. The goal is to have no significant MS activity clinically or on MRI scans. Several studies done between 2001 and 2009 have shown that conversion to definite MS from early probable MS is significantly delayed by these early preventive therapies.

Based on these rigorously conducted trials, the FDA has approved several drugs for such patients. Long-term data are even more impressive. The five-year BENEFIT trial (2009) and its eight-year extension trial (2014) showed improved outcomes in patients who started therapy early versus those who began with a placebo and then switched to the real drug when they had an MS attack. Once switched to the real drug, the placebo group improved but never quite caught up with the original group. More recently (2016), the eleven-year, long-term follow-up to the BENEFIT trial showed long-lasting, beneficial effects on disease activity, as well as improvement in cognitive functioning and the ability to hold a job.

Despite this research evidence, there has been reluctance to start treatment early by a few well-known MS centers around the country. They argue that therapy should be delayed for those patients who have a milder form of the disease until they have a significant clinical or MRI relapse. The problem with this thinking is that there is no way to predict who will have a mild disease and who won't. By the time patients with mild disease have a major relapse, it's too late to get the MS under control.

Even one millimeter of damage in the brain can destroy eleven thousand nerve fibers. A major relapse can easily destroy millions of nerve fibers, leading to a permanent disability. If you were a newly diagnosed patient with MS, would you want to take a chance to find out if you would have a milder form versus a disabling form? Studies show without any doubt that the first five years of the disease set the tone for the future course the disease may take. So, it makes sense to start the therapy early, as soon as the diagnosis is made, if not earlier. You do not want to wait until the horse is out of the barn.

Therefore, I was very surprised that this patient had not received any MS-preventative therapies. I know the neurologist who took care of Angela for two years. He is a good, caring physician, so I called him to ask about his reasoning for not starting any therapy. "Why would I want to start her on any preventative therapy? She only had two attacks!" he said. I was definitely taken aback by his response, which would have made some sense in the late 1990s and perhaps even in the early 2000s, but definitely not in 2016!

When Angela first came to see me, she was using a walker. After seven months of aggressive therapy, she is now walking without assistance. She no longer uses a walker or a cane, and she is even able to walk on her toes. Cognitively, however, she continues to remain unchanged. Perhaps her condition wouldn't have deteriorated as much as it did if she had she been put on preventative therapies at the first sign of the disease.

In all fairness to the first doctor who treated her, there are no textbook or published guidelines or algorithms for when a particular therapy for MS should be initiated, but most of the recent published literature in major, peer-reviewed journals advocates early treatment. At a time when physician burnout due to administrative overload is at record high and when a recent study in the *Journal of American Medical Association* (2016) showed that for every one hour a physician spends with a patient, two hours are spent doing administrative work, there is no time left for a physician to meaningfully learn about the latest research updates.

It is not unusual for physicians to return home from work late in the evening and spend the precious little time they have left in the day with family or even logging into the EHR from home to complete outstanding clinic work. There is hardly any time left to read journals. And even if they do have a little time, what would a general neurologist focus on—research updates on Parkinson's disease, stroke, epilepsy, MS, neuropathies, or headaches? A tremendous amount of progress has been made in all of these areas, as well as many other diseases; and to grasp all of this information would require a lot of time, which these doctors do not have.

The Value of Listening to Experts

My staff and I learn a lot within a very short time by questioning and listening to the leading experts in their respective fields who are brought to our office or present their findings at programs sponsored by pharmaceutical companies. These presentations, which are less than an hour in length, provide education that otherwise would take us months for us to learn on our own. Our physicians are able to ask questions to make sure they continue to remain on the cutting edge of therapies for their patients.

When I asked Angela's neurologist whether he had listened to visiting MS experts or attended any MS programs hosted by pharmaceutical companies, his answer was, "No. We are prohibited by our institution from attending any pharma-sponsored lectures. We are even prohibited from interacting with any pharmaceutical medical liaison or marketing personnel. We cannot accept anything from the pharmaceutical industry," he stressed.

Now, one could argue that doctors do need to keep abreast of medical advances on their own or through continuing medical education (CME) courses, as they have done in the past. But times have changed. The reality is that, given the administrative overload and the number of patients they need to see in a day, it is just not possible for doctors to keep up with research updates on their own. There has been a major paradigm shift in the last five years. Most of the physicians I have spoken to tell me how their medical journals pile up on their desk in the hope that one day they will be able to go through them. Sadly, for most, that time never comes, and the pile continues to grow higher.

This "aversion to pharmaceutical companies" started in 2007 when senators Chuck Grassley and Herb Kohl intro-duced legislation to require makers of pharmaceuticals, medical devices, and biologics to publicly report money they give to doctors. After its initial defeat, the law was reintro-duced along with the 2010 Patient Protection and Affordable Care Act (ACA) and was finally approved by Congress. This legislation, known as the Physician Payments Sunshine Act

(PPSA) and section 6002 of the ACA, requires medical product manufacturers to disclose to the Centers for Medicare and Medicaid Services (CMS) any payments or other transfers of value made to physicians or teaching hospitals. It also requires certain manufacturers and group-purchasing organizations (GPOs) to disclose any physician ownership or investment interests held in those companies, as well as any meals, honoraria, travel expenses, and grants from manufacturers.

This law mandates posting this information online in a user-friendly way for public consumption. The main argument put forth by the two senators was that shedding light on such a relationship was necessary for patients. According to an article published by *Grassley News* (2009), Kohl said, "Since we first introduced the bill, there has been a groundswell of support from every corner. Patients want to know that they can fully trust the relationship they have with their doctor."

Grassley said, "The goal of our legislation is to lay it all out, make the information available for everyone to see, and let people make their own judgements about what the relationship means or doesn't mean. If something's wrong, then exposure will help to correct it. As Justice Brandies said almost a century ago, 'Sunshine is the best disinfectant.'"

An article in the *Journal of the American Medical Association* (JAMA) (2015) underscored the value of transparency but was uncertain about its long-term effects. One of those "long-term effects" is exactly what happened to Angela. If the latest thinking that early treatment with preventive therapies is crucial, then having that knowledge could have made a difference for Angela.

The enactment of the PPSA was also influenced by the fact that, in 2007, according to a study by Eric G. Campbell et al published in the *New England Journal of Medicine*

(NEJM), 94 percent of US physicians had a relationship with the industry; 83 percent received gifts; and 28 percent received payments for professional services, such as consulting or research participation.

Furthermore, the industry paid for more than a third of all CME offerings (*Accreditation Council for Continuing Medical Education Annual Report*, 2011). How pharmaceutical-industry involvement influences doctors, research workers, and pharmacists has not been critically studied, but the implication is that the influence is "bad" and should be avoided at "all costs." To avoid press and TV publicity of the monies received, almost all universities and hospitals are now shunning the pharmaceutical-sponsored events and avoiding any interactions with their marketing representatives. The pendulum has certainly swung way to the other side from the days of mutually beneficial collaboration between the medical and pharmaceutical industries.

Transparency, as Senator Grassley pointed out, is important. But it is so not only for doctors but for every industry and for every organization. Ask any healthcare provider, and he will tell you how his patients will only get the medications their insurance companies want them to get because of the financial rebates insurance companies receive from pharmaceutical companies.

Politicians who directly or indirectly influence the delivery of medical care at a major level should also be put under the same scrutiny. In the real world, some bad always comes with some good. While the press coverage of physicians who wrongfully benefited from Big Pharma through kickbacks was appropriate and important, such coverage has created a feeling of distrust for any physician who has ties to the pharmaceutical industry. The payment of healthcare providers for their time to educate others is often thought to cause bias in their prescribing habits.

Big Pharma: A Partner in Medical Innovation

According to John LaMattina, author of two books on research and development (R&D) and the pharmaceutical industry and a contributing writer for *Forbes* magazine on those subjects, "If you go on cms.gov/openpayments and find that your doctors are being paid by the biopharmaceutical industry, don't automatically assume that they have a tainted relationship with the industry. They may instead be leaders in their fields who are looking to find the next big breakthrough to treat cancer, depression, or heart disease."

The United States leads the world in medical innovation. The ten most important medical discoveries in the first decade of this century occurred in this country, according to a large number of physicians surveyed throughout the world (ABC News, in collaboration with *MedPage Today*). The United States has the best and the most recently discovered therapies available for many diseases, as well as the latest medical technologies and breakthroughs. All of this is possible because of the close, symbiotic relationship that has existed for hundreds of years between physicians, the pharmaceutical industry, government-sponsored research, and the biomedical industry.

With the funding received from various organizations (the Office for Research Integrity in the US Department of Health and Human Services, the National Institutes of Health, the Agency for Healthcare Research and Quality, and the Institute for Medicine), Dr. Eric Campbell PhD, a sociologist and professor of medicine at Harvard Medical School and Health

Policy Research Director at Massachusetts General Hospital, conducts important research related to physician conflict of interest and professionalism. He has appeared on radio shows, is widely quoted by the press for his research, and recently testified before Congress on physician-industry relationships.

In 2004, he and his colleagues surveyed 140 institutions—125 medical schools and fifteen of the largest independent teaching hospitals in the United States—and discovered that 60 percent of department chairs had some form of personal relationship with the pharmaceutical industry. This included serving in a variety of positions, such as consultant, member of a scientific advisory board, paid speaker, officer, or member of the board of directors. At the institutional level, two-thirds of the departmental units were firmly obligated to the industry by way of research equipment, unrestricted funds, support for residency or fellowship training, continuing medical education support, and funding from intellectual-property licensing.

Is this bad? Is it unethical? We do not have any scientific studies that conclude (only imply) bias from either perspective. However, if we assume this is bad, then we must also look at the net benefit to patients and public at large. In a lifelong disabling disease that usually starts in the prime of life, such as MS, we look at the benefit of drugs versus complications, some of which could be fatal. Yet, the patient takes a chance to go ahead with therapy because the alternative is totally unacceptable. The undesirable influence of pharmaceutical companies is no doubt palpable at every level, but their contributions nonetheless are vital. It is a balance we strive for, just as we do on a daily basis with potentially fatal drug therapies.

MS, which was once considered one of the commonest causes of disability in young adults in this country, no longer has such a dire prognosis due to fourteen therapies approved by the FDA since 1993. I started to treat MS in the late 1970s. It was not uncommon then to see MS patients in a wheelchair or forced to use a walker. Now, I rarely see such patients. While there has not been a scientific study to prove this point, many senior MS experts I have spoken to agree with me that all the MS preventive therapies have made a huge difference for patients. Now, they are able to lead the lives they want to, work, and raise a family.

What is also important to note is that all these drugs were researched, developed, and brought to market by pharmaceutical companies. (No MS therapy to date has been brought to market solely by non-pharmaceutical companies). Physicians played a very important role every step of the way because they knew the disease state and exactly what would matter as far as the clinical and MRI outcomes were concerned. It also makes sense that these pharmaceutical companies, which spend upwards of $500 million (actually $2.9 billion average, according to Tufts Center) to bring one drug to market, would want to educate doctors on how to appropriately prescribe these drugs and to market them to their best advantage. And they should, to the extent allowed by law. Pharmaceutical companies use doctors who were either involved with the drug trials or who are knowledgeable about the disease state to speak to other healthcare providers around the country and the world.

Separating Physicians from Pharma

These doctors have to undergo speaker-training sessions, including the legal aspects of what they can and cannot say at these programs. They can speak only about what is consistent with the FDA-approved label; the talk has to be fairly balanced between benefits and adverse effects; and it must be accurate and not misleading in any way. Any claims made by speakers must be substantiated by appropriate FDA-approved research outcomes. Presentations have to be approved by medical, legal, and regulatory committees to ensure that they comply with FDA guidelines. The presentation slides must be presented in their entirety and in the same order as approved; speakers cannot add to or edit the slides.

Speakers are periodically audited, not only by the pharmaceutical companies but also by FDA, unannounced. They are paid according to their experience and what is considered fair market value, with a limit to what they can earn per year and per day. They take time away from their practices and their families to prepare their talks and to educate others, for which they are financially compensated by pharmaceutical companies. Speakers are required to acknowledge at the very beginning of their presentations that they are being paid by the host pharmaceutical company for their time. Despite all the restrictions imposed, one could still argue that a pharma presentation does not have the same objectivity as an independent research presentation.

Neither their malpractice medical insurance nor the pharmaceutical industry covers any legal problems that may arise related to physicians' talks. Since August 1, 2013, Big Pharma has been required to collect all data related to what they pay their physician-speakers and submit these to the proper governmental agencies. These data must be submitted annually and published in a manner that the information is widely and easily accessible by the public. This is a time-consuming, painful process requiring many hours of detailed documentation.

The names of healthcare providers, their National Provider Identifier (NPI) numbers, addresses, the food or drinks they consume at any of the meetings, any material costing over $10 (including the cost of making copies of the scientific paper) must be legibly recorded and submitted by the sponsoring pharmaceutical company to the secretary of Health and Human Services (HHS) on a quarterly basis. The penalties for failure to comply can range from $10,000 to $100,000 per payment up to a maximum penalty of $1 million.

Even though the intent of the PPSA was to ensure transparency, the repercussions of this act have produced many different reactions, one of the important ones being that a vital link in the therapeutic process is now being gradually eroded by restrictions imposed on physicians. The mandatory distancing of physicians from the pharmaceutical industry may lead to some irreparable damage that could take years to rebuild. Pharma-supported research would suffer, dissemination of information of FDA-approved drugs by pharma would suffer, and educational seminars and grand rounds at academic or private institutions would suffer.

Furthermore, the healthcare industry has changed rapidly during the last few years. Dr. Campbell's research, reported in the *NEJM*, should be directed at those who force physicians to prescribe only the drugs from which they benefit because of the financial rebates they receive and towards Congress whose members are extensively lobbied by the health-insurance and pharmaceutical industries. They are the ones who make policies that ultimately drive the healthcare industry in this country.

Even though several therapies with similar results for the same condition are approved for use by the FDA, the physician is expected to "remain neutral" and cannot be influenced by Pharma's marketing tactics, despite the fact that the physician's decision may ultimately be changed by another party who has never laid eyes on the patient. This preferential treatment to healthcare insurance companies is perfectly legal, allowing them to authorize only those drugs for which they receive significant kickbacks.

Pharmaceutical companies have a product to sell, and they want their product to be the first that comes to mind when a doctor pulls out the prescription pad and a pen, which may have the company's logo emblazoned on them. As a result of the ACA, pharmaceutical companies can no longer give out such products to healthcare providers. This is ironic because these companies can still attempt to influence physicians to write prescriptions for their drugs through ubiquitous advertising campaigns.

Recently, I was invited to give a talk at a prestigious university in California. After my presentation, residents and interns gathered around me to have an informal discussion. I knew exactly why one of the medical interns had a Band-Aid® wrapped around his pen, but I asked him anyway,

"Doctor, are you healing the pen?"

He smiled and said, "Not really. It is to hide the pharmaceutical company's logo. We are not supposed to be influenced by Pharma. We cannot attend any lectures sponsored by the industry, and we are told not to talk to the pharmaceutical reps."

I smiled but not at him. I smiled because, in the real world, it is the insurance companies that dictate what medicine our patients will or will not receive. I smiled because the honorarium I received for my talk was made possible by an unrestricted grant the university had received from a pharmaceutical company. I smiled because it was otherwise painful to see how the university was preparing its students for the real world of medical practice. Rather than educating the doctors-in-training about how to critically analyze the drug-trial studies and intelligently deal with the pharmaceutical industry, the medical establishment would instead throw out the baby with the bath water.

Preparing Medical Students for the Real World

Rather than confronting and appropriately dealing with the problem, universities across the country are simply shutting their doors to the pharmaceutical industry. In so doing, these institutions are completely missing the point. In the real world, doctors will have to face pharmaceutical reps; therefore, their training should cover how to understand research, critically analyze data, and ask the right questions. Doctors don't have enough time to read about the many clinical trials that have led to more than twenty new drugs approved by the FDA each year.

A much-quoted proverb attributed to several sources, from Chinese wisdom to the New Testament, instructs: "Give a man a fish and you feed him for a day; teach a man to fish and you feed him for a lifetime." In other words, it is better to teach young physicians to critically analyze whatever data they get from pharmaceutical companies than to simply expect them to automatically accept whatever they are told. The medical student I met in California paid a hefty sum to become a "healer" at one of our finest universities, but sadly he was "taught to apply a Band-Aid®," as he did to his pen, rather than to be prepared for encounters with pharmaceutical reps who will call on him in the future.

The imposed restrictions are beginning to have effects. Direct-to-patient advertising is on the rise. The pharmaceutical industry now spends 15,000 percent more of its marketing dollars on direct-to-patient consumers than on physician consultants. Is it preferable for patients to receive drug-related information from TV and newspaper ads than from their own doctors? While the Sunshine Act discourages physicians from giving educational seminars, it does nothing to restrict Big Pharma from advertising directly to consumers.

In 1997, the FDA allowed drug companies to market directly to consumers via public media, including television, newspapers, the Internet, and roadside billboards. This $300 billion industry spent $3.1 billion on advertising prescription drugs directly to consumers in 2012. Patients who first learn about these drugs from such media are encouraged to "Ask your doctor about [name of product]." It is not unusual for patients to shop around until they find a doctor who will prescribe what they want. This form of marketing has become so effective that drug companies are now profiting by millions of dollars in the United States and New Zealand (the only two countries where this practice is legal). I wonder what is worse: letting Big Pharma continue to interact with physicians to "educate" them on their products via sales representatives or having patients get their information from TV or other media and then seek out the therapy they want.

Those who favor direct advertising to consumers argue that these ads are truly educational. They inform patients about diseases and possible treatments. Sometimes, people suffer through problems and do nothing about them until they see their conditions acted out on TV and realize that there is an effective therapy. Ads more often encourage people to seek medical advice.

Those against such ads argue that they misinform patients and promote drugs before long-term safety profiles can be known. Prescription-drug advertising pressures health professionals into prescribing particular medications because patients want them. What people want are quick fixes; they don't worry about the potential long-term complications of drugs. Besides, they have been led to believe it is the FDA's job to make sure drugs are effective and safe to market.

The American Medical Association officially voiced its concerns and predicted the potential, serious complications of direct advertising to consumers. Seventeen years after direct-to-consumer (DTC) drug advertising was instituted in the United States, 70 percent of adults and 25 percent of children are on at least one prescription drug. According to a study conducted by the Congressional Budget Office (CBO) in 2011, the average number of prescriptions for new drugs with DTC advertising is nine times greater than prescriptions for new drugs without DTC ads. The industry now spends over $5 billion on DTC.

Internet access has made it possible for patients to go prepared for their clinic visits and to have a meaningful dialogue with their doctors. Increasingly and rightfully so, they want to participate in their healthcare choices. This is one of the reasons it is so vital to prepare future doctors to critically and intelligently interact with, rather than shielding them from, the pharmaceutical industry. It is equally important to prepare new physicians to fight for what they believe is the most appropriate therapy for their patients.

Physicians spend four years in medical school and an additional four or more in their areas of specialization before they begin their careers. Fresh out in the trenches, to survive, they have to deal with hospital administrators, health insurance companies, pharmaceutical companies, and many other agencies. Quoting Kenneth Rothman, a former *New England Journal of Medicine* (*NEJM*) board member, Dr. Lisa Rosenbaum, a national correspondent for *NEJM*, wrote, "These policies of mandatory disclosure thwart the principle that a work should be judged solely on its merits. By emphasizing credentials, these policies foster an *ad hominem* approach (attacking a person's character or motivations rather than a position or argument) to evaluating science. So why, despite such reasoned cautions, have so few been willing to listen?"

In that article, she crystalized very well the issue related to transparency, which really is at the heart of PPSA. She wrote, "No one worries about industry interacting with physicians; we worry about "corrupt industry" interacting with "corruptible physicians." Then, she asked a million-dollar question: "Are we here to fight one another or to fight disease?" I would add to that question, "Really, what disease is it that we are fighting?"

There are many diseases we need to fight and conquer, and physicians should work alongside, rather than against, Big Pharma to accomplish this. For our sakes and for the sake of our patients, physicians cannot afford to be the weakest link in that chain. We need to speak up for our patients and influence the lawmakers to bring the pendulum to a neutral position. Some important changes lawmakers should consider include ceasing to penalize physicians who abide by the FDA guidelines when they do consulting work for Big Pharma, removing all unnecessary administrative work involved in organizing seminars and educational talks, and encouraging a healthy relationship between physicians and the pharmaceutical companies.

Chapter 7

Malpractice: Taking Its Toll, Financially and Emotionally

"The greatest mistake we can make has nothing to do with missed diagnoses or medication doses, botched procedures or wound infections. The greatest mistake is to believe our worth as individuals has anything to do with any of that."
—Edwin Leap, MD

Midwest winters are always brutal. With the Arctic front moving in, the cold was unbearable. When Charles woke up at 5:00am, the temperature outside was minus 11°F. With the wind-chill effect, it was minus 40°F. It was definitely one of the coldest days on record. The National Weather Service had issued a wind-chill advisory, predicted to last for forty-eight hours, for nearly every county in southeast Wisconsin. Citizens were warned to take appropriate precautions against these life-threatening conditions; all schools in the area were closed. Before he left home to get into his car at 5:30 that morning, Charles looked in on his wife and two children, who were sound asleep in their warm, comfortable beds. His children would be asleep when he returned home from work at around 10:00pm.

The Road to Success

This had been his routine, six days a week, for the past thirteen years. But for Charles, who had grown up in northern

Wisconsin, this was his dream come true. It was not any more grueling than the six years he had spent training to be a neurosurgeon. He was elated when, after five years of hard work as a medical student, he was selected for an appointment to a neurosurgery residency program. Nothing could stop him. He had just about lived at the hospital during those years. If he got home at all, it was late at night. When he was on call every third day, the emergency and trauma center kept him busy for the rest of the night until it was time to make early morning rounds; after rounds, he went straight to the operating room.

This cycle continued without end until he became a neurosurgeon. Taking care of patients who had been shot through the spine, attending to head injuries so brutal that parts of the patients' brains protruded from their skulls, and fixing a ruptured aneurysm in the brain were all part of his life as a neurosurgeon. Learning to delicately and precisely use a scalpel to dissect a live brain, knowing that, if his incision was only a few millimeters off, it could kill or permanently damage the patient's brain—this was what made him a neurosurgeon. As the bearer of good and bad news to patients and their loved ones, then, sharing in their happiness and sorrows—this was what made him a neurosurgeon. Sacrificing his own pleasure, working long hours without a meal break, missing out on his children's milestones—this was what made him a neurosurgeon.

And now, as a practicing neurosurgeon at one of the biggest and the busiest hospitals in Milwaukee, Wisconsin, Charles felt his dream was coming true. He still worked long hours, practically living at the hospital and going home only to sleep. But he was making good money, and his life was shaping up as he had planned. He had bought a beautiful home in an exclusive neighborhood; he could afford to send his children to an elite private school; he bought the expensive car he had always wanted; and his wife could shop with a credit card that seemed to have no limit. He had started his neurosurgical career and really begun to live his life at the age of thirty-three, and he hoped to retire at age fifty-five or, at least, no later than sixty.

Charles was six years old when his father had to quit work because of the disabling effects of MS. His mother, who had never worked before, had to get a job to support three kids. His family moved from a modest house in a well-to-do neighborhood to a small apartment. All of this had a profound effect on him. The realization of the importance of money came to him very early in life. Seeing his father progressively becoming more disabled and his mother struggling to keep her job, as well as be a caregiver, haunted him even now. He had resolved never to be poor when he grew up, never to let his wife and children suffer as he had.

Growing up, Charles was greatly influenced by his pediatrician, who always came to church in a fancy car, nicely dressed in a suit and tie. Everyone seemed to know him and greeted him and his wife with respect. Charles wanted to be like this man. He observed the older man intently whenever he was taken to the pediatrician's clinic. He liked the way the doctor's assistants and nurses listened to him and the parents of sick children viewed him as supernatural—definitely not on the same level as mere mortals. He never saw anyone question the pediatrician's decisions. Not only was Charles impressed by the doctor's caring nature and ability to make sick children healthy again but also by the luxury he could afford and the power he seemed to have. Charles decided at an early age that he, too, would become a doctor. The odds, however, were against him.

* * * * *

Overcoming the Odds

Of those who are able to complete their undergraduate studies—a prerequisite to be accepted to medical school—less than 40 percent actually made it that far. According to the Association of American Medical Colleges, a nonprofit group of US schools, only 15 percent of those who desire to be doctors actually succeed. Once in medical school, it takes tremendous motivation, hard work, focus, and a competitive personality to survive the rigorous training to become a doctor. More than 6 percent of medical students drop out in the first year.

Cost is another factor that derails potential doctors. It takes fifteen to eighteen years of schooling to become a neurosurgeon; the funds required for student loans and other college costs can be very discouraging. Former Federal Reserve Chairman Ben Bernanke testified before Congress in 2012 that his son would be graduating from medical school with $400,000 in loans.

Because of his undying zeal and motivation, Charles beat the odds and succeeded in becoming a neurosurgeon. In 2003, he was recruited by a rapidly growing practice in Milwaukee. By that time, over a span of thirteen years, he had performed more than six thousand brain and spine surgeries and had received countless thank you notes for saving patients' lives. He was on staff at the biggest private hospital in Wisconsin and was admired and trusted by his colleagues and peers.

The Other Side of the Coin

But there is a dark side to practicing neurosurgery. According to Dr. Kailash Narayan, MD, program director of the neurosurgical residency at Doctors Hospital in Columbus, Ohio, "A lot of our patients are very sick, and a lot of them die or are paralyzed. The brain and the spine are unforgiving and have very little power to recuperate or heal." Neurosurgeons perform many spine surgeries on patients with chronic, disabling pain that persists despite extensive conservative therapies. Constant chronic pain makes these patients demanding, and when recovery without any significant or functional disability is not achieved, neurosurgeons become an easy target for lawsuits. Neurosurgical cases pay more to claimants than any of the specialty disciplines. In fact, neurosurgery also tops the list of specialties in the number of malpractice claims filed against physicians. It is not surprising then, that malpractice insurance premiums for neurosurgery are among the highest of any specialty, topping $300,000 a year in some states.

Dr. Ben Carson, a Republican presidential candidate in 2016, current US Secretary of Housing and Urban Development, and one of the most celebrated neurosurgeons in the world, is the author of a bestselling book, *Gifted Hands*. In his book, he describes his inspiring odyssey from his childhood in inner-city Detroit to becoming director of pediatric neurosurgery at Johns Hopkins Hospital in Baltimore at the age of thirty-three. Dr. Carson has been involved in at least half a dozen malpractice cases. Some of these cases are still pending, while others were either dismissed or settled for undisclosed amounts.

According to *The Guardian*, "His [Dr. Carson's] patients offer conflicting accounts of his near-perfect medical path toward presidential politics, describing their continued suffering from paralysis, seizures, uncontrollable bladders, and more life-altering ordeals." And yet he is a role model for many who aspire to be neurosurgeons. In his book, Dr. Carson describes how he has saved countless lives and intimately shares his struggles to beat the odds. He writes of the faith and genius that made him one of the greatest life-givers of the century.

Carson has had seven known malpractice lawsuits against him during his thirty-five-year career at Johns Hopkins. This translates into one lawsuit per every two thousand surgeries he performed. This is consistent with a study reported in the *New England Journal of Medicine* (2011), which found that almost 20 percent of neurosurgeons face a malpractice claim annually. As a consequence, some neurosurgeons refrain from operating on complex neurological problems that are at risk of developing significant persistent disability.

Others, however, recall their reasons for being neurosurgeons in the first place and do what is necessary to help their patients. Either way, the threat of being sued looms like the Sword of Damocles over them. You cannot perform more than four hundred brain and spine surgeries a year and have a perfect outcome every time. Bad outcomes are not due to deliberate or intentional actions on the part of the surgeon; but they do occur, and this keeps the lawyers busy.

Too Many Lawyers or Not Enough?

The late Supreme Court Justice Antonin Scalia observed, "...there are too many lawyers in the United States..." He went on to say, "I do not mean to criticize lawyers, just the need for so many lawyers. Lawyers do not dig ditches or build buildings. When a society requires such a large number of its best minds to conduct the productive enterprise of the law, something is wrong with the legal system."

The American Bar Association states that there are currently 1,300,705, lawyers practicing in the United States. That is approximately one for every three hundred Americans. Now, as Baby Boomers move into their sixties and seventies, and an additional fifteen million of the forty-eight million Boomers are gaining coverage and access to physician services through the Affordable Care Act, medical-malpractice lawsuits are expected to rise. To meet the new demands and to care for so many with the current number of healthcare providers, the quality of care will suffer, and mistakes will be made.

"We certainly don't expect the supply of healthcare providers to increase as fast as the demand for care," says Mark Proska, a Philadelphia-based assurance director at Pricewaterhouse Coopers. "We're anticipating anywhere from a 7 percent to 10 percent increase in the number of physicians from 2010 to 2020, compared to a much steeper increase in the anticipated growth in the percentage (36 percent) of people over sixty-five in the United States over the same timeframe. The net result would be a larger number of medical procedures being performed by a much smaller number of doctors and other healthcare providers, a condition that at least statistically increases the likelihood of an increase in malpractice claims."

* * * * *

The twenty-five-mile stretch to the hospital on that early wintery morning took Charles forty minutes. The roads were covered with ice, and as a result, traffic was moving very slowly. His first patient was scheduled for surgery at 6:15am. Normally, during his drive to work, he would go over in his mind the surgeries he was going to perform that day. But, today, his mind was occupied by something that had him very worried.

The day before, just as he was getting ready to operate, his secretary had called to say that a sheriff was at the office, looking for him and that it was important he return to the office immediately. His first reaction was that it could be something minor like being asked to be a witness in a malpractice case or maybe some parking violations. But as he started to walk towards his office, his mind raced. He thought about his wife and kids and hoped they were safe. He had seen many movies where a sheriff would be sent to a home to inform the family of the death of a loved one. He became anxious; perspiration had formed on his forehead by the time he reached his office.

He saw the sheriff holding an envelope in his hand and immediately felt relieved. It didn't appear the man was there to deliver some tragic news. After checking Charles' identification, the sheriff handed him an envelope for which he had to sign. Charles took the envelope to his office and opened it. His heart sank as he read the first few sentences. He felt faint but managed to sit down. One of his patients had filed a malpractice lawsuit against him. How could this have happened?

Charles remembered the patient. He had injured his back during a fall at work and had remained disabled and unable to work despite extensive rehab therapy, multiple pain pills, and several epidural injections. An MRI of the patient's spine had revealed a protruding disc pressing on nerves; he was told that spinal surgery could relieve some of the pain. The standard warning of any and all surgical complications, including paralysis of leg muscles, was explained to him in great detail before he signed a consent form. The surgery had gone well, but the pain had persisted. A year after the surgery, the patient was suing him for increased pain and weakness in his legs, which he felt resulted from surgery.

The Emotional Cost of Malpractice Suits

Charles was stunned. He had an intense sinking feeling in his gut—like someone had punched him. He felt nauseated and started to perspire. His extremities felt cold; an overwhelming sense of helplessness came over him. He just sat there staring at the letter. Quite some time must have passed because a nurse knocked on his door to let him know that the OR had been waiting for him for more than an hour. A quick look at him, and the nurse knew something was wrong. He couldn't admit to her that he was being sued. Instead, he offered the explanation that calls from the ER had kept him up most of the night; he just felt tired. He walked slowly to the OR to operate on a patient who coincidentally had the same kind of spinal problem as the patient who was suing him.

After the surgery, he called to notify his insurance agent, but felt greatly ashamed to mention to anyone else that he was being sued by a patient. He didn't even tell his wife.

As he drove to work the next morning, Charles was thinking about the lawsuit. No matter how much he tried to reason with himself, he felt worthless. He had done the best he could for that patient. Why was he being sued? What would his colleagues think of him? Would the suit be reported in the newspaper? What would his patients think? Would this have a negative impact on his practice and his livelihood? Once again, he felt sick to his stomach. His heart started to race.

What Charles was experiencing is not at all uncommon. An allegation of medical malpractice is extremely stressful, almost debilitating. In fact, it is one of the most stressful burdens of the medical profession. Physicians suffer from a variety of symptoms as a result of Medical Malpractice Stress Syndrome (MMSS), which was what Charles was experiencing. He could not concentrate on his work, and this bothered him. He had worked very hard all these years to become a neurosurgeon, and now he was being accused of not doing his job well. This thought kept hitting him hard. Emotionally, he was a wreck, and yet he forced himself to pretend—for others—that life was going along as usual. His work defined him. He wanted to be perceived as stoic and in command, while, internally, he was breaking into a million pieces.

It is during these stressful situations that physicians entertain the thought of ending it all, of killing themselves. Overall, the suicide rate in male physicians is three times that of the general population and, in female physicians, up to six times. The completed suicide rate (those who succeed) is the highest amongst physicians because they know what drugs to take or where exactly the gun needs to be aimed, compared to the general population. Based on a survey conducted by the AMA, an average of ninety-five medical malpractice lawsuits are filed for every one hundred physicians now in practice; and yet medical-school, residency, and fellowship programs fail to prepare physicians for such a catastrophic event.

Charles's lack of knowledge regarding legal proceedings made it even worse. He had no idea when or how this case would proceed. Later that day, he was scheduled to meet the defense attorney who had been assigned to his case by his insurance agency.

How the System Really Works

The lawyer handed him his card and reassured Charles that he was innocent until proven otherwise in a court of law. But to Charles, he had already been judged and found wanting. It was the darkest moment in his life. The lawyer went through the usual preliminaries and then talked about the lawyer who would be representing the patient. Charles recognized the name right away. The attorney's firm spent thousands of dollars advertising about how their lawyers were able to get the biggest malpractice settlement for patients. No lawyer fees need to be paid and no upfront expenses reimbursed until their clients win. The lawyer even picks up the bill for having the firm's clients examined by an independent physician of their choosing who would prepare a detailed report describing the alleged disability suffered at the hands of physician.

These medical "experts" are familiar with the legal system and know exactly what to say in their reports to obtain a favorable outcome for the plaintiff. Charles' lawyer explained that both sides would request expert medical consultants, usually from out of state. Charles's medical expert would testify that the surgery had been performed correctly and appropriately. The expert for the other side would claim the opposite—that it had been performed incorrectly and inappropriately.

Sensing how frightened and anxious Charles was, the lawyer once again reassured him that 65 percent of claims are dropped or dismissed, and most are settled before they ever go to trial. However, he also pointed out that Charles was performing over two hundred surgeries a year, well above the average for his profession. The opposite side could argue that he was greedy and performed his surgeries in haste, which then resulted in poor outcomes. Charles was shocked. While he was impressed by the homework his lawyer had done, he could not believe that "being busy" could prove to be detrimental to his case.

Charles had always been proud of how well his practice had grown and how obliged he felt to those who had referred patients him. He often stayed at the clinic to ensure that such patients were seen as quickly as possible. He spent long hours in the operating room. He worked very hard to grow his practice. Recruitment of patients was further helped by practicing at one of the busiest hospitals in Wisconsin. Never did he realize that being busy could in fact be tied to "poor outcome or quality of work." The hospital did frequent quality checks and had never informed him of any problems related to his work. No such issues were brought up when he was reevaluated for the credentialing process at the hospital. No one had ever complained about his surgical skills or the quality of his work.

"Innocent until proven otherwise" did not bring Charles any relief. For him, his patient had spoken. Even if it was only one patient, he was deeply affected. In his mind, everything positive he had ever done was negated by one bad experience, just as one drop of dye can color a whole bucket of water. He was now looking at everything with a jaundiced eye, and without question, this situation was beginning to affect his health.

In the weeks to come, Charles would turn down a number of complex surgeries and patients for whom extensive conservative therapies had failed, and surgery was considered a viable option. Instead of 6am, he began to arrive at the office at eight in the morning and return home much earlier than he usually did. He was not sleeping well and stayed up late watching TV and eating junk food. He didn't realize that the malpractice case was, in fact, pushing him into a deep depression.

Seeking Outside Support

It is during such times that physicians most need emotional and psychological support. Reassurance by colleagues that being sued does not make one a bad physician is essential. Recognizing that many other good doctors will find themselves involved in medical malpractice cases is an important step towards the healing process.

Seeking psychiatric help for major depression or disabling anxiety is also extremely important for doctors in such situations. However, many physicians hesitate to seek professional mental-healthcare, as doing so would be reported to the National Practitioners Data Bank (NPDB). The NPDB is an electronic depository of all payments made on behalf of physicians in connection with medical liability settlements, any unfavorable actions against a practitioner's license, clinical privileges, and professional society memberships. This reporting is required by federal law and is freely available to hospitals, state licensure boards, and other healthcare entities. Because this information might adversely affect being hired at another facility, physicians are obviously concerned about what is officially reported.

The lawyer appointed to defend Charles by his malpractice insurance carrier didn't actually represent Charles' interests. While he promised that he and his team would do everything possible to protect Charles, in reality, he represented the interests of the insurance company that had hired him. To avoid further expenses, the insurance company could well decide to settle the case without going to trial. Unfortunately, such a settlement would be reported to NPDB, which could tarnish a physician's reputation. It might generate questions regarding the potential competence or professional misconduct, even though the "settlement" does not necessarily reflect on the physician's competence. That's why it's a good idea for a physician to hire a personal attorney to handle any type of interaction that could result in a reportable event. This ensures that the language used in the reporting, while truthful, would be less damaging to the doctor in seeking other employment or applying for staff privileges within hospitals.

When a physician is publicly accused of harming a patient, confiding in anyone other than a lawyer or seeking guidance from colleagues is hard to do. The fear of being negatively judged keeps most doctors from reaching out for help. Support and guidance from colleagues, however, is crucial at this time. When peers repeatedly emphasize that being sued doesn't reflect on a physician's professional ability, they help relieve the feeling of panic.

Every city has strategically placed billboards and countless commercials by law firms on television, all of which encourage the public to sue and promise unrealistic financial compensation. However, I have yet to see any ads, even in medical journals or periodicals, that offer support for physicians who are being sued. In my opinion, the medical profession needs to do more to heal its healers. It has to play an active role by seeking out doctors who are being sued, providing much-needed moral support, and letting them know they are not alone. There is so much that physicians can do for one another in times of great stress. They can share stories of excellent, well-known doctors who have been sued and survived professionally; offer financial support if needed to hire a lawyer; and advise on how to minimize the negative impact of a lawsuit on their practice.

The Likelihood of Being Sued

More than 60 percent of doctors over the age of fifty-five have been sued for malpractice at least once, according to a new survey by the AMA. Although most of those claims are dropped or dismissed, the new survey from the AMA shows that most physicians will be sued for malpractice at some point in their careers.

"This litigious climate hurts patients' access to physician care at a time when the nation is working to reduce unnecessary healthcare costs," said AMA past president Dr. J. James Rohack. Malpractice lawsuits are extremely costly. The average defense costs from $22,000 to more than $100,000 for cases that go to trial, according to data in a report from the Physician Insurers Association of America. "Even though the vast majority of claims are dropped or decided in favor of physicians, the understandable fear of meritless lawsuits can influence what specialty of medicine physicians practice, where they practice, and when they retire," according to Rohack.

It takes a lot of hard work, determination, and sacrifice to become a physician. Physicians care for their patients. Their faces light up when they talk about their success stories—stories of how they pulled some patients from their deathbeds. Unfortunately, all the good they have done and do every day can be overshadowed by one malpractice case. In their minds, being sued makes them failures. It takes a toll. It affects how they will practice medicine in the future. Some become extraordinarily cautious and order more—but often unnecessary—tests just so that "everything is covered" from a legal perspective. Such "defensive medicine" (i.e., a means of self-protection against charges of malpractice in the event of an unfavorable outcome of treatment) is driving up the high cost of healthcare in this country. According to one of the largest healthcare staffing and technology companies in the United States, Jackson Healthcare, the cost of defensive medicine is estimated to be in the $650 to $850 billion range or between 26 and 34 percent of annual healthcare costs in this country.

In contrast, physician compensation accounts for only about 8 percent of total United States healthcare costs. This figure is consistent with many previous studies in finding that 80 to 90 percent of physicians report practicing defensive medicine due to fears of medical-malpractice claims. Trial lawyers who have a big financial stake in this issue aggressively fight the measure. Despite the repeated requests by President George W. Bush for a national cap on awards for noneconomic damages, such as compensation for pain and suffering or other losses not easily quantified, a proposal to accomplish this was blocked in the Senate in 2005. There were 1,143,358 lawyers in the United States as of December 2006, or less than 1 percent of the population; however, about 60 percent of US senators hold law degrees—clear evidence that this legislative body does not represent the population.

More than half of the states in this country have passed some form of a law that limits the amount of money a medical malpractice plaintiff can receive. The American Bar Association (ABA) vehemently opposes and is fighting to overturn these measures. The ABA was recently victorious in Indiana when then-Governor Mike Pence signed into law a bill increasing the payment cap. The ABA also opposes a provision that would allow judges to reduce contingent fees paid from a plaintiff's damage award to an attorney.

In Wisconsin, attorneys' fees in medical malpractice cases are limited, as are caps on the awards. Because of these measures, medical malpractice lawsuits have drastically decreased in Wisconsin. Having a cap on the award deters lawyers from aggressive marketing to recruit clients and, in some instances, from encouraging patients to file lawsuits. However, this changed as of July 2017. The Wisconsin Court of Appeals, District 1 (Milwaukee County), found the statutory $750,000 cap on noneconomic damages arising out of medical malpractice claims to be unconstitutional. The court determined that the cap was "an unfair and illogical burden only on catastrophically injured patients, thus denying them equal protection of the law."

Dr. Edwin Leap, a practicing ER doctor, in his July 2007 *Emergency Medicine News* column "Malpractice and Suicide," summarizes the issues related to malpractice very well: "The truth is, we will make mistakes. We may even cause harm. But we practice an imperfect science in an imperfect world on imperfect people. It is fraught with potential errors and disasters every day that we walk through the door to work, every time we touch a sick or injured human."

It takes a long time to heal a physician who has been sued for allegedly causing harm to a patient. Sometimes, he never heals completely. Like a string that once broken, even with the two ends tied together, is never exactly the same string. The knot remains. It is the same with physicians; malpractice claims take a critical toll, causing a trauma that may last a lifetime.

Prevention is therefore the best medicine. It is highly recommended that physicians carefully document all conversations, tests, treatments, and prescriptions. Talk to your patients, as well as their spouses, partners, or family members, about the potential risks and results. Yes, this is still another demand on your time, but if it protects you from a malpractice suit, it will be time well spent!

Chapter 8

Peer-to-Peer: The Constant Battle with Insurance Companies

"The health insurance industry does not like to pay out claims,
because they don't make money. The only way they can make a profit
is if they don't pay for your operation. If they pay for your operation and
your doctor's appointment and your pharmaceuticals,
they don't make any money."
—Michael Moore
American documentary filmmaker,
screenwriter, author, journalist, and actor

Tuesday, July 12, 2016 was like any other day at the clinic. Busy. My two mid-level practitioners and I were scheduled to take care of twenty-two patients in the clinic area, twenty in the intra-venous suite, and eight in the plasma-exchange therapy department. In addition, together we would be expected to answer more than one hundred patient calls throughout the day. To begin the day with positive thoughts and energy, we had our usual, brief team-huddle meeting.

Before I could pick up the chart to see my first patient of the day, a nurse handed me a note asking me to call the insurance company for a peer-to-peer review. This was important. The day before, I had requested an urgent MRI of brain scan for a patient I suspected had progressive multifocal encephalopathy (PML). This is a serious neurological infection of the brain caused by a virus named after Mr. John Cunningham, a native of Wisconsin.

In 1970, Mr. Cunningham was a patient at the VA Hospital in Wood, Wisconsin. While being treated with anti-cancer therapy for Hodgkin's disease, he developed rapidly progressing neurological symptoms, the cause of which could not be found despite multiple tests. He was finally diagnosed with PML after a brain biopsy was performed. Since the cause of this disease was not yet known, Mr. Cunningham willed his brain for research after his death.

Dr. Marie Gabriele Zu Rhein (University of Wisconsin, Madison) and her colleagues identified a new human polyoma virus from his brain tissue and named this virus JC, using the two initials of Mr. Cunningham's name. In patients with weakened immune systems, such as HIV infection, JC virus can invade the brain. There is no cure for this fatal infection. The prognosis is, however, a little better if the condition is diagnosed early and the offending agent causing the suppression of the immune status can be removed.

My patient, whose name was Scott, had MS, and I was treating him with a drug therapy called Tysabri, which can cause PML. Scott had received thirty monthly infusions of Tysabri and had recently tested positive for antibodies against the JC virus in his blood; this meant that he was carrying the virus in his body. The risk of Scott developing PML was estimated to be four in one thousand. The most common symptoms are memory and visual problems, behavioral changes, weakness, and seizures. We don't know the exact reason why Tysabri leads to PML, but we do know that the drug effectively blocks circulating immune cells from entering the brain. In essence, this causes an immuno-compromised status in the brain.

A few years ago, we collaborated with the Cleveland Clinic neurologists to show that, in the event that a patient develops PML, Tysabri can be effectively removed from the body with plasma-exchange therapies (PLEX). This has now become a standard therapy in Tysabri-induced PML patients. Scott had noticed a decline in his memory and new weakness on his left side. His symptoms were mild, but since he was at risk for developing PML, I had ordered an MRI of his brain to be done as soon as possible. However, according to his insurance company, he needed a prior authorization (by the insurance company medical staff) for this procedure, even though, as Scott's treating physician, I had deemed it medically necessary and urgent.

The Constant Fight with Insurers for Drug Authorizations

I dialed the number to conduct a peer review as Scott's insurance company had requested. First, I heard a recording that informed me that the conversation was being recorded for "quality purposes." Then, a live person came on the phone and asked me for the patient's reference number. After she had located the "case," she asked me to spell my patient's first and last names and tell her his date of birth. She asked for my full name, its spelling, and my telephone number in case we were disconnected. She could now see on her screen that I was calling to do a peer-to-peer review and asked me to hold while she tried to locate my "peer." Another live person picked up and asked me for the case number, the spelling of my patient's name, his date of birth, my full name, and the spelling. I was becoming slightly irritated, and informed her that I had already given all that information to the first person I had talked to.

My "peer" was abrupt. "I need to have all this information to make a decision," she snapped. I gave her all the requested information again. I wanted to know about my "peer," so I asked for her name and specialty, hoping that she was at least a physician, if not a neurologist. She told me that she was a nurse and that she would do the peer-to-peer review with me.

I asked if she was an MS-certified nurse, which she wasn't. I asked if she knew what PML was, which she didn't. At this point, I was quite irritated and impatient. I explained to her about PML and the fact that it can be fatal if not diagnosed early. I stressed that an MRI was the next important test and asked her to authorize this test for my patient. She approved the MRI "without contrast." (Administration of contrast material is necessary if you are looking for an acute inflammatory process in the brain. There is an extra cost for this). According to her, the extra money that would be spent on doing a contrast MRI was not medically necessary.

I raised my voice and asked how she could make such an important decision when she didn't even know what PML was in the first place. Once I had justified the importance of doing an MRI with contrast, she finally approved it. The whole process took "only" twenty minutes, but it definitely ruined my entire day. I was agitated and annoyed by the interaction and the time it had taken.

Unfortunately, this is not an isolated event. I am asked to do at least three to eight peer-to-peer authorizations a week, and my nurses seem to be constantly "fighting" with third-party payers for drug authorizations. This same story is taking place at every physician's clinic in this country.

The very thought of doing prior authorization invokes a negative response in healthcare providers. Not only does it kill our positive attitudes but it also makes us feel worthless to have to ask for approval from someone who usually has no understanding of the issue being discussed. While the cumulative effect of these stressful interactions on the health of physicians has not been studied, it must take both a physical and mental toll.

Dr. Mitchell "Mitch" Freedman has been practicing neurology in Raleigh, North Carolina, for more than twenty-five years. His father, who was also a physician, had instilled in him the importance of strong medical ethics. He was taught that it is a privilege to be a physician and that he should always be grateful to his patients for putting their trust in him. Mitch always puts the interests of his patients first. Anyone who knows Mitch knows too well that he will not accept no for an answer from an insurance company if he feels the treatment is necessary for his patient. Not only does he put up a vicious fight but he does not rest until the treatment is approved. Insurance companies now dread taking his calls and have nicknamed him "Tsunami Mitch."

He accepts this as a compliment. But many physicians give up or simply lack the time or resources to fight on behalf of their patients. The amount of time and manpower needed to get anything authorized for patents is getting to be exorbitant and financially prohibitive. In a study published in *Health Affairs* (2011; 30:1443-50) regarding time spent communicating with payers, researchers found US physicians spent nearly $83,000 annually on interactions with insurers, including prior authorizations. According to that study, US physicians spent an hour a week on prior authorizations, while nursing staff spent thirteen hours, and clinical staff more than six hours.

Mean Dollar Value of Hours Spent per Physician
Per Year on Administrative Costs

Personnel	United States	Canada Cost with US salaries and specialty mix
Physicians	$17,775	$9,616
Nurses	$23,478	$2,302
Clerical Staff	$37,010	$9,603
Senior Administrators	$ 4,712	$684
Overall Total	$82,975	$22,205

(Source: D. Morra, S. Nicholson, W. Levinson et al, "US Physician Practices Spend Nearly Four Times as Much Money Interacting with Health Plans and Payers than do their Canadian Counterparts" in *Health Affairs*, Aug. 2011.)

In contrast, physician practices in Ontario, Canada, spent only $22,205 per physician, per year, because of their single-payer system. That's just 27 percent of the time amount US physician practices spent. A recent online survey conducted by *Urology Times* suggests that this problem is, in fact, getting worse. Eighty-four percent of respondents report that the number of prior authorizations has increased significantly in the past two years, and an additional 14 percent say it has increased somewhat. Only 2 percent indicate that the number has stayed the same, and none say it has decreased.

Alan D. Winkler is an executive director of Urology San Antonio, the largest private provider of urological services in South Texas, which employs twenty-seven physicians and six mid-level providers. He laments, "We have to employ two full-time and three part-time employees to request prior authorizations and secure approval for a growing number of our services." Physicians do it because, otherwise, their patients would not get the necessary tests and the care they deserve.

So, who are these physicians who serve the insurance companies as "peers" to specialists? Ninety-nine percent of insurance-company doctors are family-practice physicians who have no qualifications to act as peers to specialists, such as neurologists, oncologists, and surgeons. Furthermore, they are not experienced or qualified to make decisions about requested treatments.

Insurance company-hired "peers" are not our peers. Increasingly, nurses do the work of denying requests made by medical specialists. Quite often, these "peers" cannot even pronounce the names of the drugs they have been asked to authorize. It is quite pathetic when we have to explain what the drug is for and why we want it authorized. The main goal of these "peers" is to "deny" rather than "approve." If US physicians had administrative costs similar to those of their Canadian counterparts, their total savings would be approximately $27.6 billion per year, according to the study cited above.

Bob Doherty, senior vice president of the American College of Physicians, explains the practical aspects of these huge savings this way: "It would allow each primary care physician in the United States to see another four or five patients per week, thereby reducing wait times and easing the primary-care shortage. It would increase primary-care physicians' incomes by an equivalent of $32,000 per year—more than many of the ideas for increasing primary-care pay being considered by Congress."

Why Insurance Companies Really Deny Prior Approvals

I am sure that insurance companies have their own reasons for doing what they do. Some invoke their patriotic "concerns" to declare that "it is to cut the overall health costs, which are already at record high and rising." The overwhelming majority of practicing physicians, however, do not see it that way. The decision to deny investigations or therapy, they all agree, is a business decision, rather than a medical one. The overall cost of time it takes them away from patient care, the financial and the manpower resources they must employ, and the negative impact of not getting the right therapy at the right time for their patients is far beyond any savings the insurance companies could project based on their denial of care. No one knows the patient better than his or her treating physician, so the reasoning by the insurance company "medical peers" that it is "in the best interest of patients" to avoid unnecessary tests and drug therapy is totally disingenuous.

It is obvious that insurance companies continue to use this "prior approval" tactic to maximize profits for their shareholders, as opposed to doing what is best for patients. It is simply a matter of priorities, and their priority is making money. Members of Congress, who are in position to change these practices, have not done so—perhaps because, according to OpenSecrets.org, the insurance industry spends $146,662,996 per year to lobby Congress.

Republican leaders, who have traditionally been aligned with the insurance industry, have consistently blocked any measures that adversely affect that business. Proposals that would impose liability on HMOs are denied on the basis that they would drive up healthcare costs, despite studies showing that they would be cost effective. According to a poll commissioned by the American Psychological Association and reported in *USA Today* in June 1998, 80 percent of Americans support having the right to sue HMOs, even if it means a $1 to $10 increase in premiums per month.

Why Physicians are Forced to Close Their Private Practices

Besides the huge cost associated with getting authorizations, physicians are being squeezed out of private practice for numerous reasons. Many struggle and put in long hours at work just so that they can maintain their autonomy (by keeping their private, independent practices). They sacrifice a lot in the process. More than 60 percent of physicians who own their practices say they would not consider selling, but many are forced to by laws put in place that favor large healthcare corporations.

The Affordable Care Act, ICD-10 conversion, and adoption of EHR systems are among the top issues of concern, according to a survey of more than five thousand physicians by QuantiaMD, an online physician community, and CareCloud, a cloud-based health IT vendor. Private practices cannot survive in a financial environment that supports large healthcare corporations, insurance companies, and hospitals at the expense of smaller clinics.

One of my friends was recently diagnosed with a rapidly growing brain tumor. Given the seriousness of his medical condition, it was extremely important to find the most qualified doctor in the city to take care of him. Knowing that I am a neurologist, the family called me. Before I could even suggest a neurosurgeon, they told me there were only a handful of such specialists their insurance plan would cover; the one I was about to suggest was not one of them. Up until that moment, I thought I understood what "staying within network" meant. I was wrong. What it means is that physicians who have negotiated a contracted rate with the patient's health insurance company are covered by the plan; those who have not must be paid for by the patient.

As I read through the list of permissible neurosurgeons, for the first time, I became aware of how much medical care in this country has changed in only a decade. It is now governed more by the quantity of money insurance companies make than by the quality of care patients receive. My friend needed a neuro-oncologist, but since none was listed as "in-network," he had to pay out-of-pocket to consult one. The hospital listed in his network had a general neurosurgeon but not a specialist in brain-tumor surgery, so my friend had to find another hospital to perform the brain surgery. Again, he would have to pay for this himself.

Paying these medical bills would be difficult, if not impossible. Medical debt is a huge problem in the United States—one that often leads to bankruptcy. Many of the people who incur medical debt actually have health insurance, but as in the case of my friend, the condition, the specialist, or the hospital may not be covered by the policy.

There was a time when you could easily choose the doctor you preferred, rather than having to select a complete stranger from a short list of those who have signed a contract with your insurance company. Healthcare in the United States has been transformed into an industry whose main objective to make money.

The Lack of "Peers" in Peer-to-Peer Conferences

The denial of an MRI for my patient I suspected had PML led to a "peer-to-peer" telephone conference. Now, one would think I might speak to a peer during such a phone call—a medical professional who would know what I was talking about—but one would be wrong. The majority of people assigned to these calls are primary-care doctors who are not actually peers of the specialists who order tests or treatment. Some of them are retired or soon-to-be retired physicians who are not up-to-date on the latest developments in managing highly compromised patients. Some of them are not even doctors, as was the case with my latest frustrating phone call. But frustration doesn't begin to describe our feelings when treatment choices are governed by unqualified "clerks" or nurses who override our medical recommendations.

Tremendous progress has been made in medicine over the last ten years, and quite often these "insurance doctors" are totally unaware of the drugs we request for our patients. A panel review by "experts" is sometimes convened to determine whether a particular therapy prescribed by the patient's doctor is "appropriate." This is maddening because these doctors never examine our patients first-hand and often do not even read their medical records.

Myasthenia gravis (MG) is an autoimmune disorder, which means that the body is under attack by its own immune system. Its symptoms include muscle weakness and difficulty eating, speaking, and breathing. Chase was a thirty-six-year-old man who had been diagnosed with MG about four years before I saw him. When he was transferred to our hospital in Milwaukee, he was on a respirator. He had not been helped by conventional therapies and was sent to us for advanced treatment with plasma-exchange therapy (PLEX), an FDA-approved therapy for MG. Plasma exchange involves replacing the plasma (the liquid part of a person's blood) with a commercially available protein solution.

Chase responded well to PLEX, and eventually, we took him off the respirator. After two months, he was able to speak and swallow, and he continued to improve over time. Four years later, he was down to maintenance PLEX once a month. We reduced his immunosuppressive drugs, he returned to work after a three-year hiatus, and he and his wife had a baby. He continued to improve until his insurance company suddenly denied his claims. This was based, they told me, on "evidence-based medicine"—supposedly "the conscientious, explicit, judicious, and reasonable use of modern, best evidence in making decisions about the care of individual patients." This decision, in my opinion, did not meet these criteria: It was not conscientious, judicious, reasonable, or based on any evidence of which I was aware. Again, I requested a peer-to-peer interview

My conference, this time, was with an emergency-medicine doctor who was employed by the insurance company. While he confessed to me that his experience with MG was limited (he had seen a few patients while he worked in the emergency room), nonetheless, he concurred with the insurance company's decision that Chase no longer needed PLEX.

I argued as if someone's life depended on the outcome, which, in my mind, was the case. I recited my resume, detailed my experience caring for MG patients, listed my professional designations and awards, and did everything but beg. He was unmoved. I tried to impress upon him that stopping the therapy would undoubtedly lead to a relapse. Finally, he requested that I send him all of Chase's medical records to review, which is when I realized that he had never even seen them. I was livid.

Because of this insurance company's decision, Chase missed his scheduled therapy and, within three weeks, was back to where he started. It was a worst-case scenario, including double vision, choking on liquids, and having trouble breathing. He could no longer drive or work, which meant his wife had to drive him to our hospital—a two-and-a-half-hour trip. Chase was admitted to the ICU and underwent several PLEX therapies, which were once again denied based on the same "evidence-based medicine."

The irony of the situation was obvious. While PLEX is an internationally recognized therapy for MG, and MG is a lifelong disease, Chase's insurance company ruled that it should not be given on an ongoing basis. I requested a face-to-face, peer-reviewed appeal at a much higher level and repeated everything I said before. The "peers" I spoke with repeated that the therapy would not be covered.

I called a senior neurologist at the Medical College of Wisconsin to independently evaluate Chase and to make appropriate recommendations. After seeing him, this neurologist, with more than thirty years' experience in caring for patients with MG, recommended that we resume PLEX as soon as possible. The insurance company finally approved only six therapies. At the end of those six therapies, Chase will relapse, and the fight will begin all over again.

The Tragic Cycle of Remission and Relapse in Patients Denied Prescribed Therapies

Chase's case is not unique. This happens every day to countless patients across the country, costing them a fortune in out-of-pocket payments. This is also expensive for physicians, since there is no billing code for all the time spent in preparation and meeting with insurance doctors. I can see why many doctors simply give up and let the insurance doctors make these crucial decisions, which leads to unnecessarily suffering on the part of patients. These company-hired "peers" are, in fact, making medical decisions despite never having seen the patient or, in many cases, even the medical records. They may not be medically qualified or even licensed to practice medicine in the state in which the patient lives, and, for the most part, they are not peers of the specialists whose decisions they are refuting.

Mary Corkins, founder of The Reimbursement Group (TRG), which assists healthcare organizations navigate the ins and outs of securing coverage for technology biologics and medical devices, explains why peer-to-peer is such a negative and burdensome activity: "Physician fees have been cut substantially. They are required to maintain stronger and more robust documentation of provided care. They must maintain adequate staffing, malpractice insurance coverage, re-credentialing with insurer networks, compliance with HIPAA regulations, and adherence to statutes." The impact of this continued overburdening of physicians is taking its toll, not only on physicians, but also on the healthcare options for their patients. According to Corkins, this means fewer choices and less attractive healthcare options, since physicians no longer have time to attend to peer-to peer consultations.

Chapter 9

Health Insurers' Top Priority: Profit before Patients

"I swear by Apollo Physician and Asclepius and Hygieia and Panaceia and all the gods and goddesses, making them my witness, that I will fulfill according to my ability and judgment this oath and this covenant...I will apply...(treatment) for the benefit of the sick according to my ability and judgment; I will keep them from harm and injustice."
—Hippocratic oath

I remember Sherri's first visit to my clinic thirty years ago. She was an eighteen-year-old college student who had been diagnosed with MS. She was a bright, intelligent, and very determined young lady. The diagnosis did not deter her plans to pursue her studies in apparel design and development—her major at the university. She dreamed of becoming a successful fabric designer. What impressed me most about Sherri was her positive attitude. She was motivated to succeed and ready to conquer the world. Her philosophy of life was "dream until your dreams come true through hard work and dedication." She graduated with honors in 1990 and was married two years later.

Now, at age forty-eight, she is severely disabled. Both legs are paralyzed, and she has minimum use of her right arm but manages to feed herself with her left hand. She has not stood or walked since 2005 and needs help with wheelchair transfers. Unable to control her bladder, she has a surgically installed catheter to collect urine. Since severe, painful muscle spasms in her legs couldn't be controlled with the maximum dose of oral medications, a pump the size of a hockey puck was embedded in her abdominal wall to deliver muscle-relaxing medication directly into her spinal fluid. Despite her significant disability, Sherri tries her best to stay positive and focused on her health and her marriage. The memory of how much she had wanted to be a successful professional, a wife, and a mother is painful, but she has learned not to dwell too much on her unfulfilled dreams. While her disease has dealt her a bad hand, I often wonder about the role her health insurance company has played in the progression of her disability.

More than 2.3 million people are affected by MS worldwide, with over 400,000 in the United States alone. MS is one of the most common causes of disability in young adults in this country, with two hundred new patients diagnosed each week. Within two decades of onset, more than half of all MS patients are unemployed. For Sherri, a few initial relapses were adequately treated with steroids; but in 1994, she had a major relapse that caused her to have double-vision, weakness in her legs, and an unsteady gait. Aggressive steroid and cyclophosphamide (an anticancer drug) therapy had no effect. Her condition continued to worsen until she was unable to work.

The High Cost of On-Again-Off-Again Approvals

Encouraged by our extensive positive experience with plasmapheresis therapy in such patients (including a positive double-blind randomized controlled study), we prescribed this therapy for Sherri. Unfortunately, her insurance company outright rejected our request, citing that it was not "an approved" therapy for MS patients. At that time, there were no approved therapies for someone who continued to decline, except for Betaseron, which was approved in 1993 to prevent relapses. We appealed the decision to her insurance company and provided relevant medical literature on plasmapheresis for MS.

Eventually, the therapy was approved, and Sherri began receiving treatments. Her improvement was dramatic. Her double-vision resolved, her strength and unsteadiness improved, and she was able to return to work after receiving six weekly plasmapheresis therapies. We gradually decreased the frequency of her plasmapheresis to a once-a-month maintenance regimen. She continued to do well for three years until early in 1997, when her insurance company stopped covering her treatments. Once she was off plasmapheresis therapy, Sherri began to deteriorate despite a plethora of intravenous steroids, adrenocorticotropic hormone (ACTH), and oral cyclophosphamide. Eventually, she became confined to a wheelchair.

Once again, after extensive communication with her insurance company, plasmapheresis therapy was approved in 1998. Just as before, she had a positive response to the treatment, was able to walk without assistance, and returned to work. She continued to do well with maintenance plasmapheresis therapy until early 2003, when her insurance company reversed its decision to authorize the ongoing therapy. This time, Sherri worsened dramatically and needed two people to help transfer her from a wheelchair to bed.

Treatments were eventually approved again after we pleaded with the company and shared the clinical examination videos we had recorded of her progress from day one. She improved once again with plasmapheresis and was able to walk across the hallway without assistance. However, in early June 2005, the treatments were again denied by her insurance company. This time, Sherri's condition degenerated until she became completely paralyzed in both legs. Part of her brain and spinal cord were irreversibly damaged every time she stopped therapy. In 2005, when she desperately needed her therapies, they were not reauthorized for a number of years. By the time they finally were approved, Sherri had become permanently disabled. Besides her legs, she also lost function of her right arm.

It is heart-wrenching to watch her videos, which show a severe decline every time the plasmapheresis therapy was denied by her insurance company. Over a span of twenty-three years, the decisions made by her insurance company created preventable and irreversible disability. Her dreams of becoming a fashion designer were shattered, as was her desire to have children. At this point, someone has to push her in a wheelchair, bathe her, dress her, and prepare her meals. Nevertheless, Sherri carries on with her life. When I show her videos to other physicians and medical students during educational lectures, they invoke strong emotional responses, including tears. From novices in the field to seasoned professionals, they all ask the same question: "Why? Why did her insurance companies do this?"

The Bottom Line: Profit

The answer is simple: money. Insurance companies are in business to make money. They are motivated by profit, not compassion. Patients are merely names on claim forms. Those who make these decisions never have to face real, live patients; yet, their verdicts have profound effects on patients' lives. What is so frustrating to physicians is that insurance companies are not held accountable for any wrongdoing. The government grants them immunity, which protects them from being successfully sued. In other words, insurance companies literally get away with murder.

A prescribed therapy may be denied even though it has been approved by the FDA. The decision is based not on how much good the therapy can do, but rather on how much money the company can save. The bottom line is profit, a problem that is on the rise in this country. Physicians spend an inordinate amount of time writing letters and doing peer-to-peer verbal appeals with insurance-company representatives, many of whom know nothing about the therapies they are denying. This is the number one source of frustration for healthcare providers.

Managed-care companies sell insurance by reassuring their clients that they will be covered for all necessary medical issues, based on the standards of "good medical practice." However, their definition of "good medical practice" is at odds with that of the majority of practicing physicians.

Recently, one of my patients who had aggressive MS and was doing extremely well on a once-a-month Tysabri infusion, received a letter informing him that his therapy would no longer be covered. The letter recommended less expensive therapies, even though the letter writer had never met my patient and knew nothing about him. Had that person dug a little deeper, he would have learned that all of the available therapies had not worked before the patient was finally treated with Tysabri. Nonetheless, my patient was given a choice of two of the self-injectable drugs, neither of which had been effective in the past.

I wrote a letter explaining why it would be a bad medical decision to switch from a therapy that was working to those that had not. The company sent me a reply stating that I could do peer-to-peer review; if I agreed to this, I had to give them my telephone number so that their insurance doctor could call me at a time that was convenient to him. They never agree to having a provider call the insurance company's doctors but, rather, insist on having them call us. The reason is that these doctors work part-time at different times of the day. To accommodate their unpredictable agendas, they call us and interrupt our schedules.

The following day, the insurance doctor called me at my office when I was with a patient. Normally, I do not like interruptions under such circumstances, but if I missed this call, I had no idea when—or even if—this person would call back again. Worse, yet, he might unilaterally declare the case closed, meaning there would be no more appeals!

The doctor on the phone was an internist who had difficulty pronouncing "natalizumab," the pharmacological name for Tysabri. He insisted that my patient had never tried the other MS drugs before taking Tysabri and, unless he failed all other drugs, this doctor would no longer authorize Tysabri for this patient. I was shocked. In fact, my blood pressure must have skyrocketed because I could feel strong pulsations in my head.

I collected myself and, as calmly as possible, explained to the internist the aggressive nature of my patient's MS, the medications he had failed, and that the FDA has approved Tysabri therapy explicitly for patients like this one. Furthermore, I stressed, my patient had been relapse-free for three years while he was on Tysabri. Failure on another drug meant there would be irreparable damage to his brain or spinal cord.

(One-millimeter MS damage in the brain permanently destroys eleven thousand nerve fibers.)

The doctor rejected my reasoning. The patient was switched to one of the injectable drugs and, within three months, suffered a severe relapse from which he did not fully recover. Part of his brain had died, and it would never regenerate. He became wheelchair-bound and suffered significant cognitive dysfunction. This caused a serious hardship not only for him but for his family as well. He became unemployed and lost his medical insurance. He now has federally funded insurance, which allows him to receive Tysabri once again. This process is very stressful not only to the patients and their families but also to their healthcare providers. It is stressful because we are forced to accept a therapy we know is not appropriate for our patients, and then we have to deal with the consequences.

What happened with my patient is hardly unique. I deal with such issues all the time. At every MS meeting I attend, physicians complain about how their patients are denied the therapies they require and the increasing amount of time they spend fighting the insurance companies rather than the disease. Such ongoing problems take a toll on healthcare providers. Every day, a ridiculous amount of time is wasted trying to get appropriate therapies approved for our patients. And most of the time, our prescriptions are denied for no logical reason except the financial benefit to the company.

Mind-Blowing Executive Compensation

Because they would have to cover a greater number of sicker patients under the ACA in 2016, health-insurance companies around the country sought increases in premiums of 20 to 40 percent, while several of them told their shareholders and Wall Street financial analysts that their companies would likely have higher-than-expected profits at the end of 2015.

The CEOs of the eleven largest for-profit companies were rewarded with a record-breaking compensation of more than $125 million in 2014, according to *Health Plan Week*, a trade publication. The top executives of these companies each make about $90,000 a day in compensation! For example, the total compensation for Mark Bertolini, CEO of Aetna, the nation's third-largest health insurer, was $30.7 million in 2013. This was an increase of 131 percent from 2012.

As a physician, I find it immoral for a patient to suffer from an irreversible disability due to non-coverage of a required therapy when the CEO of that very company makes in excess of $90,000 per day. For physicians, knowing how important these drugs are to our patients and what insurance company executives make each year, denial of life-saving therapies to patients is beyond painful.

As doctors, we were never trained to fight for what we believe is the correct therapy for our patients. The mismatch between what we are trained for and what we are required to do is evident. Administrative and financial management responsibilities are not discussed or addressed in medical school. Students are taught how to heal the sick. Young doctors quickly realize that the practice of medicine has become a multi-billion-dollar business, but nothing prepares them for having their medical decisions challenged by an insurance company nurse or a doctor (quite often with a different specialty) who has never laid eyes on the patient and, often, has not even read that patient's EHR.

Every state in this country requires healthcare providers to obtain licenses to practice within that state. The doctors for healthcare insurance companies, however, are exempt from the licensing requirement. It is perfectly legal for them to make medical decisions for patients in different states, without even seeing or talking to these patients. They cannot even be held accountable for any disastrous outcomes that result from their decisions.

Health insurance first emerged in the 1920s to facilitate reimbursement for the rising costs of medical care. Baylor Hospital, in Dallas, Texas, was the first to offer health insurance for a premium of 50 cents a month. It quickly became popular, and by the late 1930s, nearly three million Americans were enrolled in "Blue Cross" hospital plans. The insurance industry has continued to grow until it now controls the healthcare delivery system in this country. It has become a powerful lobby and tends to put up a huge fight whenever any legislation is introduced that might have an adverse financial effect on the industry.

These companies continue to press for higher premiums from patients, while generously rewarding their CEOs and shareholders. The amount spent on healthcare in this country every year has grown from $75 billion in 1980 to nearly $500 billion today. If this rate continues, by the year 2020, we will be spending 40 cents of every dollar we make on healthcare.

An Unconscionable Discrepancy

When a patient tells me she has had to make a choice between food or medicine or between her husband's prescription and her own, it is a story I have heard before. Across America, patients struggle to pay for their medical bills while health insurance companies earn billions. The ACA of 2010 ("Obamacare") was the most significant regulatory overhaul of the US healthcare system since the passage of Medicare and Medicaid in 1965. It was enacted to ensure that all citizens, regardless of their medical history, would have affordable health insurance.

Currently, after seven years of promising to "repeal and replace" the Affordable Care Act, Congress has been unable to fulfill that promise. Throughout all the political wrangling, the general public is left in a state of limbo, not knowing how it would all be resolved and whether they will be able to afford insurance premiums, be covered for pre-existing conditions, or lose their Medicaid. It may fall to individual states to address those concerns. The heart of the issue, however, is not primarily the ACA but rather the unsustainably high healthcare costs across the board. With or without the ACA, premiums are destined to rise if we don't change the underpinnings of the problem.

In the meantime, for healthcare providers, the most frustrating part is spending valuable time trying to convince insurance companies of the need for a certain test or therapy. This brings us back to the discrepancy between how insurance companies define "reasonable medical care" and how treating physicians define it. I have interviewed many healthcare providers who are so exasperated with the situation that they have either assumed an offensive position with insurance companies or, at the other extreme, simply given up and stopped fighting the system.

The National Institute of Neurological Disorders and Stroke lists more than four hundred neurological disorders. Years ago, we had little to offer patients in terms of effective therapies to treat many of these diseases. But in the last twenty years, science has developed new drugs, quite a few of which have been FDA approved. We now have fifteen different

FDA-approved therapies for patients with multiple sclerosis. That, of course, is the good news. The bad news is that these medications are expensive, and health insurance carriers often refuse to cover them. As a neurologist, I am all too familiar with such denials.

The Consequences of Denial of Coverage

Neuromyelitis optica (NMO) is an inflammatory demyelinating disease in which the myelin sheath of neurons is damaged, impairing the conduction of signals in the affected nerves. The five-year survival rate is 68 percent in patients with the relapsing form of NMO, with an even worse prognosis for patients who don't respond to corticosteroid therapy, the first recommended treatment. I had a patient whose optic nerve and spinal cord were affected. Her prognosis was dire. Then, I began plasmapheresis (PLEX)—a process in which the liquid part of the blood, or plasma, is separated from the blood cells, treated, and then returned to the patient's body.

PLEX changed the whole outlook for this patient. Within a few weeks, she was able to walk without help. All she wanted to do was get on with her life. Unfortunately, her insurance company denied her claim, relying on "evidence-based medicine guidelines" and insisting that PLEX was an "experimental therapy." Nothing we said had any effect on the insurance company's verdict. Our medical group routinely videotapes our patients before and after treatment to demonstrate the effectiveness of various therapies. The insurance company would not even look at our videos. Without PLEX, this patient became a quadriplegic, was put on a respirator, and, eventually, passed away.

As a result of an NMO attack, another young patient of mine became completely blind and paralyzed in both legs. Her story is similar to the first except for how it ended. With PLEX, she regained her sight, walked on her own, and went back to school. Then, her insurance company denied her claim with predictable results. Watching her deteriorate was heartbreaking for all of us. After months of holding out, the company finally relented and approved her claim. While this patient did regain her ability to walk, her eyesight was permanently damaged; she is still considered legally blind.

It is impossible to convey how infuriating it is to deal with part-time insurance company doctors who know nothing about the disease in question and have never treated anyone with PLEX. The minute such a conversation begins, we all know what to expect: months of doing everything in our power to get the decision of denial reversed.

Denial of coverage is a national pastime for health-insurance carriers. Covering expensive drugs reduces their bottom line; denying coverage improves it. It is simple math. But to cloak such decisions in respectability, decision-makers fall back on their favorite rationale—"evidence-based medicine"—a gross misinterpretation of those words. According to a 1996 report in the *British Medical Journal*, as also mentioned above, the phrase "evidence-based medicine" was intended for "the conscientious, explicit, and judicious use of current best evidence in making decisions about the care of individual patients."

It's amazing how that simple definition has been twisted to provide an excuse for insurance companies to deny claims. According to an unsubstantiated report, supposedly written by health insurance companies, at least 20 percent of treatments prescribed by doctors must be denied if the industry is to remain profitable. That percentage appears to be accurate. The National Nurses Organizing Committee reports that from 2002 through 2009, six of the largest insurers operating in California rejected 47.7 million—22 percent—of all claims. This is an average. The committee reported that during the first half of 2009, insurance company PacifiCa did its part to double that statistic by denying 39.6 percent of claims. Cigna, HealthNet, Kaiser Permanente, and Blue Cross were all well over 20 percent. Only Aetna was below this figure.

The insurance industry was quick to deny these figures, but as a treating physician, I would say these numbers are right on the mark. And I am not alone. Physicians across the country, as well as some of my patients who cannot afford to pay for ongoing treatment, would certainly agree. Those who can afford to pay in the early stages of treatment may lose everything they have as their medical expenses escalate. In 2013, CNBC predicted that "...bankruptcies resulting from unpaid medical bills will affect nearly two million people this year—making healthcare the number one cause of such filing."

Pre-Existing Conditions + Higher Copayments + Increased Premiums = Bankruptcy

According to a study by the American Society of Clinical Oncology (ASCO), cancer patients are three times more likely to declare bankruptcy than those with other diseases because they are not told what to expect. "Most doctors do not discuss the potential costs of treatment with patients," said Marilyn Marchione in a report on KCCI 8 Des Moines. "Many doctors are not having the conversations that might help prevent (bankruptcies) and sometimes don't know the cost, themselves." Dr. Rahma Warsame of the Mayo Clinic, who led the ASCO study, observed that this would not occur in any other industry where a service or product is sold.

Other unexpected expenses result from the denial of coverage of pre-existing medical conditions or charging exorbitant amounts with higher copayments—two ways insurance companies make money. If the insured person gets sick, his premiums are dramatically increased, making them difficult to afford. Even if the insured person remains healthy, his premiums continue to increase each year. I have yet to hear from any of my patients that their premiums have decreased!

For healthcare providers, the other major problem is delayed payments or outright rejection of claims, even when the rendered care was preauthorized. Insurance companies are allowed to reconsider their decision to cover a particular illness or therapy and then deny payments. In such cases, unfortunately, physicians have no recourse.

One would think that abortion is the only issue of concern to politicians; it certainly is the only one they talk about. But there are others of equal importance that the health-insurance lobby prevents Congress from addressing, including the soaring cost of drugs, CEO salaries, the focus on profits over patients' welfare, and the acquisition of private medical practices by insurance companies and hospital systems.

The industry also controls which FDA-approved drugs will be covered by insurance and which will be denied, a constant game of musical chairs. There seems to be no discernible reason a certain drug is considered "preferred" one year but not the next, since no new studies have demonstrated any difference in efficacy or side effects. Based on statements by a number of drug-industry officials I have interviewed, these decisions are based on "rebates received," which is another way of saying "kickbacks." Existing laws have made the practice of receiving rebates and restricting drug choices legal, widespread, and growing.

The industry has taken its invincibility one step further by appointing independent "pharmacy business managers" (PBMs) to negotiate on their behalf. As in the approval of certain drugs, PBMs are also driven by rebates. The higher the rebates, the greater the chance of a drug being listed on the company's drug formulary. It takes a significant amount of time and valuable resources for a physician to convince insurance-company personnel that the prescribed non-formulary drug is in the best interest of a particular patient. Sad to say, they are often immune to such arguments.

Congress has passed laws that make these practices not only legal, but also acceptable. And Congress has the power to change those laws. What is preventing them from doing so are the deep pockets of three powerful lobbies. The pharmaceutical and health-products industry, which includes not only drug manufacturers, but also dealers of medical products and nutritional and dietary supplements, hit a record of nearly $272.8 million in lobby spending in 2009 when the ACA was being debated in Congress. The American Hospital Association's total lobbying expenditures in 2016 were $22,117,895, and total campaign contributions by the health insurance industry were close to $10 million. (Source: OpenSecrets.org). That money buys a lot of influence, and it's hard to imagine members of Congress turning their backs on this largess.

Absence of Legal Guidelines to Ensure
Fair Pricing of Drugs

One place this influence can be felt is in the rising cost of drugs. For example, the yearly cost for any of the fifteen specialty drugs approved for MS ranges from $60,000 to over $150,000. According to the National Center for Health Statistics, the total national health expenditures for 2013 were $2.9 trillion, of which 9.3 percent was for prescription drugs. Even though more than four out of five prescriptions in this country are filled with generics, the rising cost of specialty drugs contributed to a 3.2 percent increase in total prescription drug spending to $329.2 billion.

The *MS Institute for Healthcare Informatics Report on Prescription Drug Spending* revealed that spending on prescription drugs in the United States rose 12 percent in 2015, mostly fueled by new and costly drugs for cancer and hepatitis C. Spending on treatment for autoimmune diseases rose by 28 percent to $30.2 billion.

Progress in medicine has led to decreased mortality and morbidity, largely because of the pharmaceutical industry's investment in research and drug development (R&D). Even though the industry continues to make huge profits, those profits are proportionally matched by the amount spent on research. Overall sales and marketing expenditures were about $30 billion in 2016, versus about $150 billion in R&D costs. It should also be noted that companies in virtually every industry spend more on marketing than on R&D. That said, biopharma ranks number one on R&D investments.

However, there are no legal guidelines to ensure fair pricing of drugs. Pharmaceutical companies are at liberty to charge what they feel is "reasonable" based on the efficaciousness of the drug. Drug pricing is soaring as a result. The price of older drugs is also rising every year. The cost of preventive injectable drugs for MS approved by the FDA in 1993 and 1996 used to be under $11,000 to $12,000 per year. The same drugs are now priced over $50,000 to $96,000 per year. This reflects an increase by 30 percent per year over the last twenty years!

Recently, we have witnessed a handful of pharmaceutical companies, which have invested very little in research on drug development, buy drugs (from the original inventors of the drugs) when their patents expire and drastically increase the price of these drugs. For example, in 2010, CORE Pharma bought a lifesaving drug, Daraprim (used in the treatment for malaria and toxoplasmosis), and increased its price by more than 1,200 percent. However, this absurd and unethical act received little attention until Turing Pharmaceuticals bought the same drug in 2015 and raised the price by an additional 5,500 percent. While this price jump was perfectly legal, it attracted a lot of negative national and international publicity.

Despite pushback by medical professionals and patients, the price of the drug was not lowered. The 2016 Democratic Party presidential candidate, Hilary Clinton, took advantage of the publicity it created and tweeted that she would introduce a plan "to combat the issue" of pharmaceutical price-jacking. She did not get the chance to follow through on her promise. The CEO of Turing was eventually arrested, not because of the dramatic and irrational increase in the drug price, but for some other unrelated reason.

Unexplained drug price increases are a common practice among the pharmaceutical companies. The price of Cycloserine, a drug used in the treatment of drug-resistant

tuberculosis, was increased from $16.66 to $360 a pill. Vale-
ant Pharmaceuticals, a manufacturer of two heart drugs—
Isuprel and Nitropress—increased the cost of their pills by
525 percent and 212 percent, respectively. Doxycycline, a
commonly used antibiotic for many years, recently went from
$20 to $1,849 a bottle.

Immediate decisive pushback by the Biotechnology
Innovation Organization (BIO), the world's largest trade
association, resulted in termination of Turing Pharmaceutical's membership. BIO cited that Turing's leadership did not
reflect the commitment to innovation and values that are at
the core of BIO's reputation and mission. Censorship by such
organizations and government-sponsored hearings to address
these unscrupulous tactics are a step in the right direction.
However, since the practice of drug price-jacking remains
perfectly legal, patient advocacy is an uphill struggle. Physicians are caught between efforts by organizations like BIO
and the pharmaceutical and health-insurance industries,
which are the nation's two highest financial contributors to
politicians.

According to *New York Times* columnist Nicholas Kristof,
the drug industry spent $272,000 in campaign donations per
member of Congress in 2015. Kristof reports that there are
more drug-company lobbyists than members of Congress. It
should be no surprise that complaints by healthcare providers,
who are already under pressure, continue to be ignored.

How to Get Prescribed Therapies Approved

The guidelines below are offered by Dr. Elliot M. Frohman,
MD, PhD, FAAN, a world expert in MS and one of the greatest patient advocates I know. While his suggestions may not

ensure adequate authorization of the therapies being prescribed, they tilt the scales in your favor and provide the
comfort of knowing that you have done everything possible to
care for your patients.

Dr. Frohman advises that you begin any conversation
with the insurance company doctor by introducing yourself
and stating your affiliations, your specialty, and any recognition awards you may have received. Then, ask for the insurance industry doctor's name and specialty, what states he is
licensed in, and if he is still in practice or retired.

If authorization for the therapy you have prescribed is
denied, make the following statements: *If you deny the
requested therapy before we get off the phone ...*

- *From now on, you will co-manage this patient with me.
  Welcome aboard. I'll add your name and contact information to the records so that all notes can be sent to you.*

- *I will also embed your name and photo in the patient's
  electronic health records.*

- *Of course, I will document your refusal to approve my
  recommendations for the management of my complex
  patient, even though you've never seen, examined, or met
  him.*

- *If my patient is denied treatment and his condition
  deteriorates, I will help him document what was done or
  not done to cause his adverse outcome. I will share the
  responsibility with you for failing in our fiduciary duty to
  provide the right treatment for my patient's specific
  disease. I have obtained my patient's consent to have this
  conversation and to communicate our shared intentions. If
  you hang up, all of the above will be immediately implemented.*

Dr. Frohman claims he has been successful in obtaining the appropriate therapies for his patients 100 percent of the time, which is an amazing track record. He insists that insurance companies can and will approve the correct therapy if they are challenged. His method is certainly worth a try.

What we really need are laws that prevent insurance companies from denying life-saving therapies for no other reason than profit. That is the job of Congress, which is, unfortunately, in thrall to the powerful insurance lobby. The question is: *What would it take to break that grip?*

Chapter 10

Physician, Heal Thyself:
How to Restore, Replenish, and
Rejuvenate to Beat Burnout

"If physicians aren't happy, they can't heal others."
—Vivek Murthy, MD, MBA,
the 19th Surgeon General of the United States

This book describes all of the daily frustrations endured by physicians—frustrations that are creating a burnout crisis in the medical community. But my message wouldn't be complete if it didn't propose solutions to this crisis. In writing this book, I have tried to positively empower physicians to fulfill our mission: to better advocate for our patients, to care for our patients with compassion, to take a stand against what is not right, and to change our own lifestyles to heal from within.

The solutions I offer are based on my own experience and that of hundreds of physicians I've had the privilege of meeting and talking to around the country. My colleagues and peers have personally benefited by adopting the changes and solutions outlined in this chapter. The point I want to make is a simple one: There is no art to practicing corporate medicine, which is so mechanical and devoid of compassion that it turns physicians into assembly-line workers. For the welfare of our patients, for the art of medicine to flourish, and for our own survival, we need to fight back by healing ourselves and finding strength in our collective power. In short, we must organize.

By "organize," I mean the following: as physicians, we must come together and marshal our resources in order to form decentralized, legal entities to provide compassionate healthcare services that promote health and recovery.

How to Deal Effectively with Administrative Power

If you want to change your life, change your thoughts.

Nothing kills your body and the soul as much as negative thoughts. It's easy to tell you to stay positive, but I know how difficult this can be when you are working under stressful conditions. Here are some recommendations you can try if you truly want to change your thoughts.

- Celebrate the fact that your years of hard work, focus, and sacrifice were made possible by your determination to care for and heal others.

- Resolve not to feel let down by unreasonable demands to which you are subjected.

- Do not give in to intimidation.

- Remind yourself of these encouraging words by a medical pioneer, Sir William Osler: "To have striven, to have made the effort, to have been true to certain ideals—this alone is worth the struggle."

- Look at this problem from a physician's perspective: Positive thoughts can boost your immune system and your health to help prevent "burnout."

Become proactive.

Think beyond the walls of your workplace. Many other physicians are experiencing the same things you are. To bring about positive changes in the healthcare industry, we have to cultivate public awareness of the problems faced by physicians and share that information, particularly with our patients.

Patients can be a powerful catalyst for change. Make them your partners in correcting these problems. Every chance you get, let them know the facts and how the present situation is having a negative impact on the kind of care they receive.

Be vocal. Write to the media, and encourage them to report all of the ways that current practices are affecting you and your patients. These detrimental policies and regulations have been put in place by Congress and corporate healthcare organizations. Make your patients aware of these policies. The public has a powerful voice that can be effectively harnessed by physicians. However, this force needs to be awakened.

We need to earn people's trust and foster their confidence in us. We need to galvanize the public across the country to work with us to change the way healthcare is managed and delivered in this country, and we need to change the perception that physicians are responsible for the high cost of healthcare.

Play an active administrative role.

Since there is a real need to recoup costs, there is nothing wrong with having business-minded administrators in healthcare systems. But as physicians, we have a responsibility to ensure that patients are not harmed. Healthcare policies should be developed by physicians and executed by administrators, not the other way around. It is the duty of local medical societies to advocate and speak up for physicians. Private-practice doctors can join a labor union as individuals, but we are prohibited by law from bargaining collectively over our salaries, benefits, or working conditions.

The United States is in the minority of all industrialized nations in which doctors are not allowed to bargain or negotiate collectively. However, some unionization has occurred in this country, the most notable being the Union of American Physicians and Dentist (UAPD), which was formed in 1972 and was an instant success because of the frustrations physicians were facing at the time. Many other unions were formed throughout the country, but almost all of them were short-lived.

When our hands are tied, unions can be our most powerful ally. Why, then, have unions not succeeded? There are many reasons, including the interpretation of union laws and the legality of such unions being successfully challenged in the courts. The health maintenance organization (HMO) industry condemns what it regards as doctors' efforts to circumvent the antitrust laws.

However, one of the most important reasons unions didn't succeed is described by Grace Budrys in her book, *When Doctors Join Unions* (1997). "Doctors are bad at taking a collective stance," Budrys writes. "They are slow at taking actions to challenge their new and dissatisfying conditions at work." Budry concludes with a prediction that physicians are now at the threshold of taking a stand. She has no doubt that doctors will take action in response to their growing resentment about being moved closer to employee status and further from the decision-making center. "How soon they decide to take more aggressive steps remains to be seen. How effective doctors are when they do take action will vary, as well. However, no one should be surprised to learn quickly from each other's successes and failures."

Take care of your own.

I am not referring here to "burnout programs" for physicians, which play a crucial role in every institution. I am talking about reaching out your hand to your peers who are in need, lending them your ear, and showing compassion for your fellow physicians when they are going through a rough time.

Speak out against any injustice you may witness. Form ad hoc committees to collectively raise concerns, if speaking out alone is not in your best interest. Listening to well-recognized medical professionals talk about the prevalence of this problem nationally, as well as locally, will broaden your perspective and help you deal with it on a practical as well as an emotional level.

Being connected with other physicians around the country has a powerful therapeutic effect. Coping with the problem alone is difficult; sharing it with others and finding strength in numbers is the first step in solving it.

Focus on patient care.

Focus on patient care, rather than spending your time trying to satisfy performance measurements and process improvement metrics, which do very little to improve physician-patient relationships. If these policies are mandatory at your institution, then ask administrators how they actually improve patient care.

If patients were asked their opinion about the care they receive, they would be quick to point out the endless procedural steps they are required to undergo and how little time they spend with doctors. Physicians should be compensated not only for time they spend with patients but also for the hours they devote to paperwork, fielding phone or email questions, and doing complicated coding. This would allow them more quality time with patients and lead to appropriate financial compensation.

End the silent struggle with stress.

Your brain and your body react adversely to demands put on you. If the demands are unpleasant, unrewarding, and demeaning, they can affect your physical and mental health. Let us face it; you cannot get rid of many of the stressors you face in your daily life. You can, however, react to them in a positive way. You can choose how to react to stress. You do not have to become a victim. You can fight back. There are three proven ways to fight back the ravages of stress: *restore, replenish, and rejuvenate* (RRR).

Restore

Restore your health and vitality by exercising. Shed the excess weight, and trim down to fight back, to do what you worked so hard to achieve. Thirty minutes a day is all it takes to take care of yourself. This should be a piece of cake compared to the grueling hours you spent to become a doctor. Do it now. Do it for yourself, do it for your loved ones, and do it for your patients.

As discussed earlier, obesity is a medical crisis in this country. It has overtaken smoking as the leading preventable cause of cancer in the United States. According to a report published in *The Scientist* (2015), even a modest decrease in weight can reduce the risk of cancer. Several possible mechanisms have been suggested to explain the association of obesity with increased risk of certain cancers, according to the National Cancer Institute (NCI).

Exercise can dramatically reduce cardiovascular diseases. New research discussed in the American Heart Association's journal, *Stroke* (2016) shows that people who were declared physically fit in their mid-forties, had a significantly lower incidence of stroke after the age of sixty-five, independent of traditional stroke risk factors, such as high blood pressure, type 2 diabetes, and atrial fibrillation.

Exercise can improve your emotional well-being. Research done at Duke University showed that thirty minutes of brisk exercise three times a week was better than Zoloft, an antidepressant of the selective serotonin reuptake inhibitor [SSRI] class for treating depression! According to Duke psychologist James Blumenthal, the effectiveness of exercise seems to persist over time if you continue to do it. (*Journal of Psychosomatic Medicine*, October 2000).

Replenish

As physicians, we encourage our patients to maintain a healthy diet. We should focus and make a conscious effort to eat healthy as well. We know the consequences of being overweight. Eating well and exercising regularly helps prevent obesity. It is not only important to eat less, but also to drink lots of water! Rule of thumb: Drink one large glass of water (222 ml) for every 22 pounds of body weight a day. Drinking two 222 ml glasses of water before every meal can lead to twenty-two pounds of weight loss a year. Furthermore, one of the commonest causes of fatigue is dehydration. Being dehydrated by 3 percent can decrease your strength by 19 percent.

What should your caloric intake look like? Determine your caloric intake by multiplying your current body weight by 12 to determine the number of calories you should take daily. You need 0.5 to 1 gm of protein per pound of your body weight (20 to 35 percent of all calories), less than 25 percent of calories from good fats (such as those found in avocados, flax seed oil, olives, nuts, and fish oils), and the rest from carbohydrates (whole grains). It is better to eat more smaller meals, which include one-sixth of the total protein you need. Whey proteins, when accompanied by exercise, improve exercise performance, body composition, and biological markers of health (*Medicine & Science in Sports and Exercise*, December 26, 2013).

Avoid any kind of soda, including diet soda.

Soda may be comforting and convenient to drink, especially when you are under physical or mental stress. There is now ample scientific evidence to show that chronic consumption of diet sodas actually promotes weight gain (*Metabolism: Clinical & Experimental*, 63: 69-78, 2014). Even though non-nutritive sweeteners have no calories, a study from Oita University in Japan showed that mice fed with water with non-nutritive sweeteners increased blood sugar levels far more than those fed with water with no non-nutritive sweeteners. The mice who received non-nutritive sweeteners, gained body fat and increased leptin and triglyceride levels.

Avoid cigarette smoking.

More than one-third of all doctors in China and Italy smoke cigarettes. In the United States, while that number is declining, it is estimated that 5 percent of doctors smoke. This is roughly about 50,000 physicians. One of every five deaths in this country each year is due to cigarette smoking. It is the number-one risk factor for lung cancer, accounting for about 80 to 90 percent of all lung cancers. Tobacco smoke is a toxic mix of more than seven thousand chemicals, many of which are poisonous. At least seventy are known to cause cancer in people or animals.

The main way smoking causes cancer is by damaging our DNA, including key genes that protect us against cancer. Now, researchers have, for the first time, identified the organic compound acrolein (acrylic aldehyde), which is released while smoking cigarettes, as highly cancerous. In a large study reported in *BMJ Specialty Journals* (September 2005), smoking just one to four cigarettes a day almost triples a smoker's risk of heart disease and lung cancer and creates a 50 percent higher risk of dying from any cause than non-smokers. Smoking is by far the biggest preventable cause of cancer and other serious medical problems. Research has shown that for every fifteen cigarettes smoked, there is a DNA change, which could cause a cell to become cancerous.

Take supplements, including Omega 3.

Some of the important supplements to consider are vitamin D and Omega 3. Vitamin D is actually a pro-hormone because the body is capable of producing its own using sunlight on the skin. There are two major forms, D2 and D3. D3 is approximately 87 percent more potent in raising and maintaining twice to three times greater storage of vitamin D than is D2. A review of more than fifty vitamin D studies also shows that vitamin D3 offers a noticeable decrease in overall mortality.

In a double-blind, randomized study (2016), Vitamin D3 significantly improved heart-muscle function in people with heart-muscle weakness. Vitamin D3 selectively regulates certain genes and the immune system. New genes are being discovered every day that vitamin D either up-regulates (increases the cellular response to a stimulus) or down-regulates (decreases the cellular response to a stimulus), and many immune cells have receptors for Vitamin D. It is also important in regulating cell growth and synaptic communication between cells, and may reduce cancer progression.

After reaching a desired blood vitamin level (usually sixty to eighty ng/ml), an average adult man requires 4,000 IU of vitamin D3 daily to sustain the desired level.

Polyunsaturated fatty acids reduce inflammation, control hunger, switch off fat genes, and moderate blood sugar. The National Institutes of Health (NIH) recommends 1,600 mg of Omega 3 daily. Omega 3 fatty acids can increase the myelin content of motor nerves and improve motor-skill performance.

Take one-a-day multivitamins.

Doctors Kathleen M. Fairfield and Robert H. Fletcher of the Harvard Medical School in Boston, Massachusetts, recommend that all adults take a daily multivitamin. Their two-part report appeared in the June issue of the *Journal of the American Medical Association* (*JAMA*, 2002). Fairfield and Fletcher reviewed studies published between 1966 and 2002 of relationships between vitamin intake and various diseases. They concluded that sub-optimal levels of vitamin intake are associated with an increased risk of contracting a variety of chronic diseases, including cancer and heart disease.

A more recent Harvard study (*Journal of Nutrition*, 2016) revealed that when men used a daily multivitamin for at least twenty years, they had a 44 percent lower chance of heart attack and stroke (cardiovascular disease) than those who did not use a daily multivitamin for the same timeframe. This an important finding as heart disease is the leading cause of death among men in the United States. It is estimated that one in every four males will die due to heart disease. The American Medical Association now recommends taking a multivitamin pill daily.

Take probiotics for your gut microbiome.

In our gut reside around 100 trillion organisms, which compose something called our "microbiome." For every one of our cells, there are ten microbial cells living on or inside our body, which are crucial to our health and survival. Recent research discovered differences in gut microbiota composition between healthy and diseased individuals. "Unhealthy bacteria" in the gut promote inflammation, in contrast to the healing properties of "good bacteria."

Many different disease states (e.g., auto-immune inflammatory, degenerative, and cardiovascular disorders; cancer; and obesity) have been linked to an altered intestinal microbiome. Emerging preliminary data provide a hint of the health benefits of replacing bad bacteria with good. According to a new meta-analysis published in the *International Journal of Food Sciences and Nutrition*, consuming probiotics (so-called "good" bacteria) can reduce body weight and body mass index (BMI).

Get more sleep.

"Sleep is the best meditation," writes the Dalai Lama. According to the Centers for Disease Control and Prevention, between fifty and seventy million adults in the United States have a sleep or wakefulness disorder. The issue is so large scale that it is considered a public health problem. Sleep deprivation leads to a stressful state, illness, and accidents.

Adequate sleep at night (between seven and nine hours) reduces the production of hormones that could increase appetite. Sleep deprivation slows your metabolism, while increasing your appetite.

You should feel refreshed after a good night's sleep. If you don't, something is wrong! Sleep deprivation also can upset your emotional equilibrium. Recent studies headed by David Dinges and his group (2012 to 2017) show that sleep deprivation lowers your threshold for handling stress, explaining why some people becoming enraged over small annoyances.

The myriad demands put on physicians (e.g., work pressure, deadlines, needing to complete EHRs, etc.) cause them to cut back on their sleep. The resultant stress may lead to health risks such as obesity, diabetes, high blood pressure, coronary heart disease and stroke, poor mental health, burnout, and even early death.

So, what can you do to sleep better? There are some important habits that can improve your sleep health:

- First, recognize the importance of sleep, and resolve to get the recommended seven to nine hours of sleep every night. Even one night deprived of sleep has noticeable health consequences the following day.

- Be consistent. Go to bed at the same time each night and get up at the same time each morning, including on the weekends. If you have difficult falling asleep at the desired time, consult your physician to see if a short-term sleeping pill is recommended to re-establish your circadian rhythm.

- Restrict the use, or better still, remove all electronic devices from the bedroom.

- Avoid large meals, caffeine, and alcohol before bedtime. Get into the habit of exercising on a regular basis. This can help you fall asleep more easily at night.

Rejuvenate

Try yoga and meditation. Chronic stress is like a poison that kills you slowly. It alters the status of your immunological and physiological state to promote inflammation, increases the incidence of cardiovascular disease and cancer, and causes memory problems. The practice of daily meditation helps reduce the effects of chronic stress.

In a study of people over fifty-five years old (in whom the brain is, perhaps, less plastic) who practiced one hour of yoga weekly and twelve minutes of meditation daily for three months, there was a significant improvement in memory and mood, as well as a reduction in anxiety. Meditation also has a profound effect on the autonomic nervous system, which controls all bodily functions, including the immune system. With mediation, such as mindfulness (a mental state achieved by focusing one's awareness on the present moment), you can positively and consciously influence this system to your advantage.

In his best-selling book, *Anatomy of an Illness*, Norman Cousins spoke to our current interest in taking charge of our own health. He wrote that "(the) greatest force in the human body is the natural drive of the body to heal itself, but that force is not independent of the belief system. Everything begins with a belief."

We are born with a genetic "blueprint," and for many years, it was believed that our bodies grew and developed according to this blueprint without our ability to change the outcome. In other words, our fate was immutable. This no longer reflects current thinking. In spite of our genetic blueprint, we can most definitely take action to stop or alter many diseases once they occur.

How can genetics be changed? The science of epigenetics is proving that our environment and choices can influence not only our genetic code, but also that of our children. Both positive and negative thoughts have a profound effect on genes. The most recent research now confirms that proper nutrition, exercise, and de-stressing our bodies can also modify our genes.

Take-away Message

To avoid or to counter burnout, your intention should be to attain and maintain optimum health. To do so, follow common-sense health and fitness principles:

- Eat consciously and selectively.
- Meditate fifteen minutes a day.
- Get seven to nine hours of sleep.
- Exercise daily.
- Stay hydrated; drink at least eight glasses of water a day.
- Spend just a few moments each morning deciding to make it a great day.
- Maintain an attitude of gratitude. Spend a few minutes at the end of day jotting down the things that went well that day and that you are thankful for.
- Appreciate your colleagues; help them when appropriate or necessary.
- Challenge administrators if you disagree with them, for your patients' and your own well-being.
- Leave your workplace at a decent time so that you can enjoy the rest of the day doing what you like to do.
- Acknowledge that getting angry kills you and no one else!

Practice the Most Powerful Medicine—Kindness

- Start your day with meditation, prayers or some sort of reflections to invoke a positive state of mind. Understand that it is a privilege to serve your patients, who put their trust in you.
- Always be positive while interacting with your patients. The love and energy you receive in return will do wonders for you and your health.

- Get to know your patients' work and their families. Having this information goes a long way toward healing your patients.

- Frustrations will occur. Dealing with EHR, administrators, and health insurance will be stressful. Recognize that you are doing all of this for your patients. If you do not fight for your patients, no one else will. They are your top priority.

- Do not be controlled or governed by issues that do not improve patient care.

"If you are not ready to alter your way of life, you cannot be healed."

—Hippocrates, a Greek physician who developed an Oath of Medical Ethics (460BC–377BC)

Minimize the Chances of Being Sued and Know What to Do if You Are

Spend more time with patients.

Do not rush. The quality of medical care improves when you are not juggling too many things at once. Patients and their families appreciate being adequately attended to by their physicians.

Dr. Wendy Levinson, a professor at the University of Toronto, published a very important study in the *Journal of American Medical Association* (*JAMA*, 1997). She and her colleagues studied more than 1,200 conversational behaviors of fifty-nine primary-care physicians and sixty-five surgeons—some who were never sued and some who had been—with their patients. They concluded that the most important reason patients with bad outcomes sue their doctors is not medical negligence but rather how their doctors interact with them. Listening, paying attention, addressing their concerns, and having open and honest communication markedly reduced the risk of litigation.

Many other similar studies have come to the same conclusion. The decision to take legal action is determined not only by the original injury but also by insensitive handling and poor communication after the original incident. In other words, communicate clearly and effectively and be sure that you are understood.

Make a personal connection with your patient.

Do it even if you are required to use a computer in the examining room. This is critical. EHR plays a very important role in patient care, but it also creates a multitude of problems. However, the practice of medicine is rapidly changing. The mandatory use of EHR makes it very difficult to have a personal connection in the short time you have with patients. Twenty minutes for a follow-up and forty-five with a new patient are the new norm. It is also important to remember that the EHR records the total time you spend with your patient. A hurried visit can be held against you. This is a tough juggling act to master. On the one hand, you are pressed to see more patients in a short time, and on the other, you are supposed to spend quality time with your patients. Reschedule the patient for another visit as soon as possible if you feel you don't have sufficient time.

Apologize if you make a mistake.

Many studies have shown that if a doctor expresses a genuine concern for the injured and apologizes for errors, the patient or grieving family is less likely to file suit. Some hospitals now have a professionally trained risk-management team that proactively works with an "injured patient" to minimize the risk of litigation.

If you are sued, inform your family, colleagues, close friends, and the hospital. The ten physicians I interviewed who have been sued at least once completely agree with this advice. The emotional support they received, especially from their peers, was extremely beneficial. If you know a colleague who is being sued, reach out to that person. Give as much emotional support as possible. Call or text your colleague to let the person know you care.

Call your local medical organizations hotline for support.

Request help from someone who is qualified to handle an emotional conversation with a distressed doctor. In addition, if your hospital has a team of professionals who can meet with you on a regular basis—not only regarding emotional issues, but also to make sure that your reputation is not damaged— by all means, make an appointment. If this service is not available, then talk to your attorney to see what proactive measures you can take to avoid any damage to your professional reputation.

If the suit is published or discussed in the media, the best approach is to work with the hospital to give a truthful and appropriate response to the press. If there has never been a quality-related issue raised about you in the past, point that out to your hospital administrator. Be proactive.

Retain your own attorney.

Your personal attorney will help you manage all the information that will have to be reported to the National Practitioner Data Bank (NPDB). Remember, your malpractice insurance attorney has no vested interest in your case because he is employed by the insurance company.

The Role Hospitals and Clinics Must Play

The commonly held belief that doctors can take care of themselves is totally false, especially in the current healthcare environment. The problem of physician burnout, however, is a recent phenomenon. Traditionally, physicians would approach any problem by looking for its underlying causes. Only then would they be able to propose a solution. While it is well known that the principal cause of physician burnout is administrative dominance, finding the best solution is complicated.

How can hospitals and clinics successfully address this problem when their administrators are the primary cause? How can we expect clinic and hospital administrators to proactively diagnose physicians who are heading toward burnout or are already there, when the administrators themselves are in large part responsible for that burnout?

This is not an impossible scenario. Here are some things that hospitals and clinics can do to help:

- Establish wellness programs exclusively for physicians. These programs should involve a psychiatrist who is trained to recognize and mitigate burnout.

- Hold regular meetings with small groups of physicians and encourage them to vent their frustrations freely and safely with no negative repercussions. This is key to their engagement.

- Gently confront physicians who are obviously heading towards burnout or are already experiencing it, knowing that physicians are notorious for neglecting their own mental and physical health. Once they are aware of it and know they have support, they are more likely to seek help.

- Your appreciation and expression of concern may actually be the best medicine.

The Role Physicians Must Play

What I have offered here are some short-term solutions. What is needed, of course, are long-term or permanent solutions; but even if we find them, we are not likely to implement them without changing the environment in which we work. This will be difficult, but I believe it is achievable. While Congress is heavily influenced by lobbyists who are more focused on making money than on achieving a fair and a balanced healthcare system for all, physicians have an important role to play in solving this problem.

- First, we need to voice our concerns to our local elected officials—to start with influential people in our communities with whom we can actually meet face to face.

- Then, we must begin to collectively fight for our rights and insist that our voices be heard. As physicians, we are not used to doing this, but it's time to wake up from the dream that the situation will somehow magically change. The reality is that it will not change unless we change it.

- As uncomfortable as it may feel at first, we need to assert our power, not only for ourselves but also for our patients. Patients are victims of the same upside-down healthcare system we are attempting to change. Our fight is their fight, and we must be the conduit for their message to reach lawmakers.

- The bottom line is that, as physicians, we must unionize! I am aware that current laws do not favor this solution, but laws can be changed. Congress can be influenced. Lobbies can be defeated.

- We are at a watershed moment in terms of healthcare. If we do nothing, the art of medicine as we have known it will simply cease to be. The corporate entities that have turned the care of the sick into profit-making ventures will change the face of healthcare, possibly forever. That is a high price to pay for doing nothing.

- On the other hand, if medical providers stand together to fulfill our mission, we can preserve the art of medicine. We can care for the sick as we were trained to do. We can prescribe state-of-the-art therapies without interference. We can eliminate the time-consuming, stress-producing clerical duties that have nothing to do with patient care. We can spend more time with our patients, listening to them with compassion and using our experience and intuition to correctly diagnose their illnesses.

- On a personal level, we can restore our self-confidence and dignity. We can enjoy our work instead of dreading it. We can take back our careers and our lives. That is our prize for taking action.

Chapter 11

Good Karma: The Most Powerful Antidote to Anger and Despair

"The best way to find yourself is to lose yourself in the service of others."
—Mahatma Gandhi

Words are dynamic. They evolve over time and change to reflect the culture in which they are used. "Karma" is such a word. The Hindu and Buddhist concept of karma is what will happen to you in your next life based on what you do in this lifetime. In scientific terms, karma is a law of nature that you reap what you sow. In everyday parlance, this same idea is expressed as "what goes around, comes around."

Nowhere is this idea as obvious as it is in environments in which so many physicians now work. These workplaces range from fast-paced and stressful to downright toxic. All that negative energy is as contagious as any disease. A physician who is overworked and overburdened by administrative work is at risk of taking those negative vibes and sending them right back out again. On the receiving end will be medical and office staff and, worst of all, patients. Let me give you an example that is very close to home for me.

My sister, Bena (not her real name), who lives in Texas, had a good relationship with her primary-care doctor for a number of years. The doctor always took her time when Bena went for her check-ups, inquiring about family and work. In the past, the visits were upbeat. However, Bena noticed a gradual change in her doctor's behavior and that of her doctor's office staff over the last five years. She couldn't remember when she first became aware that everyone seemed so rushed. No one had a spare minute for conversation. In fact, both nurses and doctors spent most of their time typing on computers, which they brought into the examining room.

The Boomerang of Bad Karma

Bena's doctor no longer seemed interested in how my sister's family was doing or what was going on in her job. This was upsetting to Bena. She trusted her physician and looked up to her, but the doctor's attitude had changed so dramatically, she was almost a different person. Instead of asking, as the physician had done in the past, "How are you feeling?" or "Is anything new going on?" the doctor asked, "What is your problem?" without making eye contact. Then she did a quick scan, ordered tests, wrote a prescription, and hurried out of the room.

Bena was crushed. She felt humiliated by her doctor's treatment. The end of this story is not unusual; in fact, it is becoming increasingly common. My sister left the office and never returned. Sadly, her physician of many years did not bother to follow up to ask why.

Of course, not all stories end that way. If we do indeed reap what we sow, it's a good idea to pay attention to what we are planting. I'm happy to report that many doctors do just that. Here is an example of one doctor who planted a veritable garden. I had accompanied Anu, my youngest sister, to the hospital for a major surgery: a total left mastectomy. She had been diagnosed with breast cancer less than a month after her husband passed away of a sudden heart attack at work.

Anu's tumor was quite large on her initial ultrasound, but the latest MRI showed that five months of hormonal therapy had shrunk it by 90 percent. It was now time to remove the breast. Despite Anu's terrible peripheral veins, the process of starting an intravenous line went extremely well that morning. She received some of the preoperative medications, and we were waiting for the surgeon to meet with us before she was to be wheeled into the operating room.

Receiving the terrible news that she had cancer, while grieving the loss of her husband, had been rough on her. Following the diagnosis, she had been given daily blood-thinning injections in her stomach to alleviate the thrombosis of the jugular vein in her neck, which was caused by the placement of a catheter to administer her anti-cancer drugs. She also received daily hormonal therapy to combat the cancer.

It is at times such as these that we all need someone to turn to for comfort and encouragement. Sometimes, it is a family member or friend; sometimes, it is our faith in God or a higher power. When we are in trouble and someone comes forward to help, the weight is lifted from our shoulders, and we feel that we are not alone. We experience a sense of relief and hope. But, when there isn't a "someone else," an unexpected sign is often enough.

Anu found her sign the first time she went to her husband's office after he passed away. She needed something that would bring order to the thoughts racing through her mind, some signal to give her strength to continue with her life. She had closed her eyes for just a moment, and when she opened them, she saw a penny at her feet. She picked it up and read the words, "In God we trust." She found the sign she was looking for!

The Ripple Effect of Good Karma

While we were waiting for the surgeon to arrive, my sister-in-law, who had come to wish Anu well, handed me a small framed picture of Ganapati, the elephant-headed Hindu god of wisdom and learning, as well as the remover of obstacles, and asked that I put it under Anu's pillow. As I was wondering how to fulfill that request, the surgeon arrived to talk to us. Just as she was about to leave, I said, "Dr. Mikkelson, we have a favor to ask of you but would totally understand if you decline." I showed her the picture I had in my hand. "Would you mind keeping this with you during the surgery?"

"I am honored that you would ask me to do this," she said. "I can certainly use the guidance this God will provide, and I will pin it to my pocket while I am operating on Anu. It always helps to put your trust in God." I was totally surprised by her response, for it was not the way most surgeons would have answered.

After the surgery, Dr. Mikkelson came to see us, and as she removed the picture from her pocket, she gave us the good news. "The surgery went really well, and the lymph nodes she had removed were all free of cancer!"

In the next few days, I kept thinking about Dr. Mickkelson's response to my request and the words she had chosen to convey her feelings. It reminded me of Maya Angelou's famous saying, "I've learned that people will forget what you said, people will forget what you did, but people will never forget how you made them feel."

This doctor had given Anu hope when she so desperately needed it. But, even more importantly, her words spoke of her self-confidence and the joy she obviously derived from healing and soothing others.

As Francis of Assisi said more than seven hundred years ago, "For it is in giving that we receive." There couldn't be a better example of "good karma."

Remembering Our Mission

In these rapidly changing times, when physicians are under pressure from every direction and the burnout problem is at a record high, a conscious effort to remind us of our mission to our patients may just be what we need. Giving is powerful. It invokes a variety of changes in our immunological and neurophysiological systems to promote self-healing and wellbeing.

Mahatma Gandhi and Winston Churchill, two of the most iconic figures of the twentieth century, were arch-enemies. They never saw eye to eye on anything. They fought each other bitterly. Gandhi was trying to gain Indian independence from Britain, while Churchill was trying to preserve the British Empire. But they both agreed on one thing: the importance of giving.

Churchill once said, "We make a living by what we get, and we make a life by what we give."

Gandhi said, "It is not what and how much you give; it is the manner in which you give that is important."

We reap what we sow. What we send out into the world is returned to us in kind. When we are angry, it seems that everyone around us is angry. When we are smiling, other people smile back at us. Our actions produce effects that are not only returned to us but also ripple out farther than we can imagine.

Physicians touch so many lives every day—people who are suffering, people who need help. A gift of a simple, uplifting gesture can do wonders, sometimes even more than a prescribed medicine could accomplish. The interesting thing is that such an act also does wonders for the physician. There is no scientific study to prove this, but I have heard this idea echoed by so many physicians. Essentially, what they are saying is, "My patients keep me going; they are the ones who make me want to come to work when everything else looks so bleak and depressing."

Loving care and a genuine concern for patients creates a good feeling, which, in turn, sends positive energy back to doctors. Using functional MRI, numerous studies have shown that the brain's pleasure areas are activated by acts of kindness. Giving or receiving an act of kindness gives us pleasure and happiness, which creates positive physiological changes, causing the donor to receive far more than she has given. Kindness has a soothing effect on the cardiovascular, emotional, and immunological systems.

Barbara Fredrickson is a professor in the Department of Psychology at the University of North Carolina at Chapel Hill and Director of the Positive Emotions and Psychophysiology Laboratory. Her pioneering research suggests that cultivating gratitude in everyday life is one of the keys to increasing personal happiness. "When you express your gratitude in words or actions, you not only boost your own positivity but [other people's] as well," she writes in her book *Positivity*. "The beneficial effects of fostering an upbeat emotional attitude are being extensively studied. Positive psychology is an emerging science that focuses on how your emotions and your actions can influence not only you but the people you interact with as well."

Training the Brain to Be Happy

Richard Davidson, a neuroscientist, is a professor of psychology and psychiatry at the University of Wisconsin-Madison, as well as founder and chair of the Center for Investigating Healthy Minds at the Waisman Center. He has spent nearly forty years studying the human brain and emotion. Applying the latest MRI technologies to his research on Tibetan monks has shown that cultivating compassion and kindness through meditation affects brain regions that can make a person more empathetic to other peoples' mental states.

According to Davidson, "Just as exercise can turn a flabby stomach into a six-pack, mental training, such as meditation, can fine-tune the brain and, consequently, your emotional style." The brain is plastic and in a state of constant change. Thus, it can be trained to overcome the damage created by burnout. Davidson has shown that people can learn to increase activation in the areas of the brain that cause happiness and to suppress those which invoke negative emotions.

For a physician who is overworked and overburdened by administrative work and who sees his revenue diminishing, it takes learning and a conscious effort to stay positive. The amount of paperwork doctors have to do in addition to caring for their patients is not only stressful but is also one of the principal factors leading to the emerging burnout crisis in the medical community.

The recent research showing that the physician burnout rate in this country is at a record high came from Mayo Clinic. During a TV interview on WTTW in Chicago, Dr. John Noseworthy, CEO of the Mayo Clinic, advised patients to fire their doctors if they suspect physician burnout. While I can understand my sister's decision not to return to her physician, for a CEO of the most premier medical institute in the world to suggest such an action is not helping physicians. If patients heed his advice, many of the physicians at the Mayo Clinic and nationwide would be fired.

This would be a catastrophe when the pool of active physicians is in decline. CEOs and politicians make decisions, which on paper may make sense, but in the real world of medical practice, do not. To understand what physicians do every day would require these decision-makers to walk a day in their shoes—to experience in real time what doctors are expected to do on an hour-by-hour basis. This is probably the only way they would grasp the impossibility of these expectations.

Stopping Burnout in its Tracks

Since that is unlikely to ever happen, we physicians must address the burnout crisis on our own. That is a tall order. It begins by asking ourselves some tough questions, such as, *Am I more tired at the end of the day than I used to be? Do I feel as if I'm on a treadmill every waking hour of the day? Has work taken over my life not because of dedication but because of decree? Have I lost control of my own practice? Am I thinking of quitting?*

These are the symptoms of burnout, and they are danger-ous. If you asked yourself these questions and answered yes to most of them, that's a red flag. What can you do to turn the situation around?

First, you should focus on why you became a doctor in the first place. Wasn't it to put patients first and ensure that their care superseded all the administrative and clerical demands thrown at you? Here is one such simple example. At my clinic, we use EHR, and despite many hours of training, I still find it horrible. Inserting some orders is frustrating and takes a long time, so instead of getting "mad," I now write the orders the old-fashioned way—by hand. I would rather spend that valuable time with my patients, and I want to be in a cheerful mood when I am with them. The administrators of my clinic insist that I then go back and enter my orders into the EHR.

My priority is my patients. Patients trust their doctors with their lives. They look up to us and seek advice on many issues, and they place us above any other professionals they deal with. They feel demeaned when they get short shrift and rude treatment from burned-out physicians. Their trust is shattered. The trauma (and I use that word advisably) they experience takes a long time to heal.

The second thing physicians should do is understand the consequences of stress. Chronic stress at work can cause many health problems for physicians as well as their patients. Suzanne C. Segerstrom authored a meta-analysis report, based on three hundred articles, that described the relation-ship between psychological stress and the immune system. (*Psychological Bulletin* 2004 Jul; 130(4): 601–630) The report concluded that chronic stressors are associated with suppres-sion of both cellular and humoral immune systems, making physicians more vulnerable to illness and disease.

Invoking positive thoughts or showing kindness to others has just the opposite effect on the immune system and, subsequently, on health. Michael J. Poulin, associate professor of psychology at the University at Buffalo College of Arts and Sciences, tested 846 participants and confirmed the hypothesis that providing help and kindness to others contributes to reduced stress and mortality.

The Positive Power of Neurotransmitters

We have known for centuries that giving to others makes us feel good, which releases neurotransmitters, such as endorphin, oxytocin, serotonin, and dopamine, in our brains and, in turn, motivates us to do more productive work. The feeling lasts over time, and we now have a scientific evidence to prove it. A stressful situation causes cortisol and adrenaline to be released into our system, leading to a "fight-and-flight" response, which ultimately weakens our defense mechanisms to fight infection and other diseases.

A display of positive quotes in patients' rooms and in our offices helps to draw us back into the caring, giving mood. It is easy to get so wrapped up with the day's hassles that we neglect to return to our spiritual zone.

I learned this lesson and many others from a patient—let's call her Annie—who was dying from a severe attack of MS in her brainstem. The attack left her completely paralyzed from the neck down and dependent on a respirator to help her breathe. Even the very aggressive therapies I tried failed to produce any improvement in her condition. During her forty days in the ICU, I spent a lot of time with her. Our time together changed my life. I believe she helped me to become a better physician.

Each time I came to examine her, Annie would focus all of her attention on me, trying to help me understand what she was feeling. What I saw in her eyes was determination. She was not about to give up the fight. It was hard to forget the expression in her eyes, which stayed with me long after I left the hospital each day.

Annie was a massage therapist. Her passion was helping people relax and feel better. The first time she came to my office, she was using a walker. She immediately told me, "I will go back to work one of these days."

Though Annie's condition continued to deteriorate, she was always cheerful and quick to tell a joke when she visited the clinic. My staff and I enjoyed seeing her; her positive attitude was contagious. I had first seen her in 1984; only six years later, I found myself having to tell her about the seriousness of her condition. I had spent some time preparing what I would say. I took her hand in mine and began. "Annie, the damage to your brain is permanent. What that means," I explained, "is that you will be on a respirator for the rest of your life. You will not be able to talk, eat, or move your arms and legs again. Your mind, however, will not be affected. It will as sharp as it is now.

"Do you understand me?" I asked. She nodded her head slightly to say yes. "While you are here with us," I continued, "should your heart stop for any reason, do you want us to do all we can to get it going again or let nature take its course?"

She looked at the nurse, who knew that she wanted her alphabet board so that she could answer my question. As she blinked her eyes to indicate the letters, the nurse spelled out, "If my heart stops, I want a heart and lung transplant."

Healing the Patient's Soul

Annie was not through fighting. I had done everything medically possible to heal her body, but medical science has its limitations. Her eyes haunted me. They were always trying to tell me that she needed something else from me. On my way home one evening not long after that conversation, I got off the highway, turned around, and went back to the hospital. I walked to Annie's room, gently put my hand on her head, and asked, "Are you scared? Are you afraid to die?"

On her alphabet board, she spelled out "Y-E-S."

There was nothing to say. My mentor had once said to me, "If you can't do anything to save your patients, then at least hold their hands and be there." So that's what I did; I held her hand and stayed. Having no idea how she would respond, I asked if she would be willing to have a priest spend some time with her. She nodded.

When Father Joe entered her room, he said, "Doctor, go home. I will talk to her."

Father Joe called me at home that evening to assure me that he had a long talk with Annie and she was at ease. A few hours later, Kathy, an ICU nurse, called and said, "Annie passed away in her sleep."

I did a lot of thinking that night. Not for the first time, I realized that there is more to treating patients then ordering lab tests, diagnosing illness, and prescribing the newest available therapies. I was fortunate to have someone to teach me the importance of holding our patients' hands and reading their eyes. I knew I had done everything possible to treat Annie's disease, but understanding what she was trying to tell me with her eyes was more difficult. I felt that it had taken me too long to get her message.

Annie's soul needed to be healed before she could let go. As a physician, I was attempting to heal her physical being, while Father Joe was able to calm her soul. That is not something I had learned in medical school, and I doubt that young physicians are learning it now. But it is perhaps the most important lesson we can learn from our patients.

As we begin to address the myriad problems causing physician burnout and strive to find solutions, focusing on our patients, understanding their unspoken needs, and simply holding their hands will be a step in the right direction.

Acknowledgments

I want to thank all my colleagues who have shared their stories of frustration, anger, and despair with me. It would have been impossible to write this book without their stories.

I would especially like to recognize Bobbi Linkemer, who once again did an outstanding job as my editor. She drew from her own experience as a patient and interactions with her healthcare providers in getting the best out of me. She asked appropriate questions, made excellent suggestions, and nudged me ever not so slightly if I slacked off, all of which made this a better book.

I also want to thank my teacher and mentor, Dr. Michael P. McQuillen, for reviewing all of my chapters, for his suggestions, and for keeping me updated with stories related to physician burnout published in medical journals and newspapers.

I owe a debt of gratitude to my family, Radovan Stojanovich, and to all my brothers and sisters who offered not only criticism but also encouragement and motivation to continue.

Many thanks to my co-publisher, Kira Henschel, for her calm patience with me and for her knowledgeable guidance; to Peggy Nehmen for her brilliant cover design; to all who recognized the importance of what is being said in this book and for writing powerful testimonials; to Joe Sweeney for his excellent foreword; and to anyone else I may have inadvertently omitted.

I appreciate all that you have done to make this book a reality. Thank you!

About the Author

Bhupendra O. Khatri, MD, is the founding medical director of one of the largest multiple sclerosis centers in the country. He has been honored by the National MS Society with a Lifetime Achievement Award and is consistently rated by peers and patients as one of best neurologists in Milwaukee, Wisconsin. Dr. Khatri lectures nationally and internationally on caring for patients with neurological disorders and on the power of the subconscious mind on healing.

In his best-selling first book, *Healing the Soul: Unexpected Stories of Courage, Hope, and the Power of Mind*, he became the voice of his patients and their caregivers as they coped with the devastating effects of MS and other serious neurological conditions.

Now, as then, he fears that the art of medicine is under threat from lawmakers, regulators, insurance companies, technology, and hospital administrators. In this new book, *Healthcare 911: How America's Broken Healthcare System Is Driving Doctors to Despair, Depriving Patients of Care, and Destroying Our Reputation in the World*, he expresses the frustrations and fears of medical providers across the country who are experiencing unprecedented emotional and physical strain created by these factors.

For more information, please visit Dr. Khatri's website:
www.KhatriMD.com

Index

Abbreviations ACA, EHR, ICD, MS, and PML stand for Affordable Care Act, electronic health records, International Classification of Diseases, multiple sclerosis, and progressive multifocal encephalopathy, respectively.

219

hospital mergers, 19–22
"Hospitals Firing Seasoned Nurses:
    Nurses FIGHT Back!" (newspaper
    article), 19
human growth hormone (HGH), 102
human polyoma virus, 142
human right, healthcare as a, xi

I

insomnia. *See* sleep/sleep deprivation
Institute for Critical Infrastructure
    Technology (ICIT), 45
International Classification of
    Diseases (ICD)-9, 66–67
International Classification of
    Diseases (ICD)-10
    as a mandatory requirement,
        65–68
    administrative demands, 66, 73,
        83–88
    changing medical practice, 71–73,
        82, 149
    coding as a hospital asset, 68–70
    diagnosing illness, 83
    reimbursement, 68–71
    See also electronic health records
International Diabetes Federation, 96
*International Journal of Food Sciences
    and Nutrition*, 186
International Journal of Obesity, 93
"iPatient," diagnosis and treatment, 42
Iraq War, combat casualties, 51–58
Isuprel (isoproterenol), 172

J

Jackson & Coker (medical recruiting
    agency), 8
Jackson Healthcare, 138
James, William, 103
JC virus infection, 141–43
Johns Hopkins Hospital, 93, 127–28
Journal of Nutrition, 185
Journal of Psychosomatic Medicine,
    181
*Journal of the American College of
    Surgeons*, 62
*Journal of the American Medical
    Association* (JAMA), 36, 111, 185,
    190
Jurca, Radim, 96

K

Kaiser Permanente (insurance
    company), 167
Kandel, Eric, 103
Karl, story of lifestyle and exercise,
    89–93, 102
karma, good vs. bad, 197–202
"kickbacks." *See* rebates/kickbacks
kindness as medicine, 189–90, 202–3,
    206
Kohl, Herb, 110–11
Kristof, Nicholas, 172

L

LaMattina, John, 113
Landstuhl, Germany, 52
lawyers. *See* attorneys/legal
    representation
Leap, Edwin, 139
Levinson, Wendy, 190
license/licensure, 26, 135, 153–54,
    162–63, 173
lifestyle and exercise
    attitude and motivation, 89–92,
        175–80
    benefits of, 101–4
    caloric intake and diet, 181–83
    cigarette smoking, 183
    finding the time for, 101
    overcoming burnout, 95–101
    restoring health through, 180–81
    sleep/sleep deprivation, 186–87
    story of Asish Trivedi, 97–104
    story of Karl, the bodybuilder,
        89–93
    vitamins, supplements and
        probiotics, 184–86
    See also obesity
Liu-Ambrose, Teresa, 104
lobbying and buying influence, 81,
    117–18, 148, 168–69, 172, 194–95
Lublin, Fred, 106

M

malpractice, lawsuits/insurance
    ACA and increasing claims of, 129
    being sued, the likelihood of, ix,
        137–40, 190–93
    giving up private practice, 22–23
    insurance company exemption, 76

220

CPSIA information can be obtained
at www.ICGtesting.com
Printed in the USA
FFOW02n1854200218
45151221-45704FF